INTERMITTE
FOR WOMEN OVER 40

Lose Weight, Detox Your System, Increase Your Energy, Reset Your Metabolism and Rejuvenate Your Whole Body includes a 7 Day Kickstart Weightloss Plan.

BY

Amanda Clarke

Disclaimer:

All information in this book (including text, graphics, and others) is only for educational purposes. Adequate efforts were made to present accurate, up-to-date, reliable, and complete information in this book.

Under no circumstances will any blame or legal responsibility be held against the publisher, or author, for any damages, reparation, or monetary loss due to the usage or application of the information in this book, either directly or indirectly.

The book is not intended as a substitute for professional medical advice, diagnosis, or treatment. Always seek the advice of a qualified healthcare professional regarding your medical condition. Never disregard professional medical advice or delay in seeking it because of what you read in this book or elsewhere.

If you think you may have a medical emergency, please contact your healthcare provider immediately. Any mention of products or services is not intended as an endorsement, recommendation, or guarantee of such products or services or the company that provides them. Any information provided in this book is used at your discretion and is solely at your own risk. Please discuss your best options with your healthcare service provider.

TABLE OF CONTENTS

INTRODUCTION

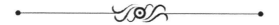

Intermittent fasting can be described as periods of voluntary abstinence from food and drink. This type of fasting is not a new idea as it has been in practice since ancient times, and it is also discovered to have tremendous benefits on the body and brain. Some of such benefits include changes in weight and metabolic parameters associated with type 2 diabetes, cardiovascular disease, and cancer.

This book aims to provide an overview of Intermittent Fasting programs and give important necessary information about the health benefits, especially in relation to needs of women over the age of 40 and focusing on the benefits that Intermittent fasting can provide for them. The majority of information about Intermittent Fasting currently is obtained from research in animal models. Hence, critical studies in rodents are briefly summarized.

This Book also provides a detailed explanation of the relationship between fasting and human health in general.

It reveals the connection between Intermittent Fasting and circadian biology, gastrointestinal microbiota, and modifiable lifestyle habits such as food, activity, and sleep.

In this Book, we will talk about various intermittent fasting regimes and what you need to know about them, especially for women over 40.

Enjoy!!!

CHAPTER ONE

WHAT IS INTERMITTENT FASTING?

Even if fasting at intervals or intermittent fasting sounds almost outrageously novel, the opposite is the case. Like many other diets, interval fasting is a recurring phenomenon. In simple language, Interval fasting means nothing more than "interrupting" fasting in various ways. It is not a diet, such as a diet consisting of low carb or low fat, but the oldest form of nutrition that humans know.

In practice, it involves alternating periods of food intake and fasting. The Interval model is done based on the daily routine of hunters and gatherers. After all, before the so-called Neolithic Revolution, man spent much of the day chasing animals and collecting all kinds of berries, fruits, and nuts.

In reality, there was never space during this period for constant food consumption, as is the case with our modern societies. The people only had time to eat food in peace when the "loot" returned to the village. Intermittent fasting is, in theory, the most efficient form of the human diet, which is especially useful due to its simplicity of execution.

What Differentiates Intermittent Fasting from Religious Fasting and Other Diets?

In intermittent fasting, we don't talk about the distribution of macronutrients or certain foods' renunciation. This is because, at this point, the interval leaves you more or less free, in that respect. It is a basic system, as I have said, with quite simple rules that you can tailor to your individual preferences or requirements and as such, there are no explicit rules except for an existing calorie deficit. Of course, you should try to eat foods that are balanced and rich in proteins. However, if you design fasting at intervals with a leaning towards a low carb, low fat, or high carb diet, it is up to you.

Religious fasting, such as the one practiced in Islam during the fasting month of Ramadan, is quite different from intermittent fasting. Intermittent fasting is about configuring fasting windows and liquid, while in Ramadan, the strict interpretation also prohibits fluid intake. With some exceptions, you can drink as much as you want during fasting periods during intermittent fasting. The only requirement, however, is that it should be drunk without calories and that it that should be a clear liquid such as water.

CHAPTER TWO

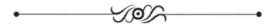

THE BENEFITS OF INTERMITTENT FASTING

Intermittent fasting has some critical advantages over other diets. This refers to, among other things, the hormonal environment for burning fat. The decisive starting point here is that blood sugar levels do not rise gradually during the day due to the short periods of food intake; it also increases insulin sensitivity in the body. At the same time, it releases the anabolic growth hormone HGH. The conclusion is that it optimizes the biosynthesis of proteins and consumes fat.

Research also shows that this diet can protect cells in the body against oxidative stress and free radical harmful effects. It has also been shown that fasting cycles can lower LDL cholesterol levels by activating nerve cells and positively impacting cognitive performance. This is not all there is to its numerous benefits. Another value is that you don't have to think about sticking to strict nutritional schedules or explicit diet bans and nutrient hours all the time. Interval fasting is an optimal diet and allows you want to eat enough despite your diet. Suppose you want to participate in celebrations, eat at a restaurant, or visit your friends without significant restrictions. In that case, all that is needed is proper time management to get the correct windows.

What Are the Disadvantages of Intermittent Fasting?

There is no perfect method anywhere, and that also applies to extended fasting. Of course, to be efficient with this system, you also need to consider certain drawbacks from the very outset. Unless you feel that you can survive without games, then you're mistaken. The fasting time is only half as adequate without strength training and supplementary endurance activities. There's nothing in here, even without a predominantly healthy diet. Occasionally junk food is permitted, but it may not be scandalous. So, with that principle, you don't get a free pass to celebrate.

One of the most significant drawbacks is also on the psychological side. You should get used to not feeding for several hours if you are used to eating several times a day. The chance of enjoying the epigastrium's agony, also known as hunger pain, is solid in the early days. On the other hand, intermittent fasting is not recommended for those who have already overcome an acute eating disorder because conversion will exacerbate an eating disorder. Due to the sharp decrease in blood sugar levels, the fasting interval is also not suitable for people with diabetes.

As an original form of human nutrition, fasting at intervals is not far from our internal conditioning. Consequently, the potential for weight loss success is excellent. And those hundreds of thousands of people have already demonstrated that the method works. If you want to get rid of body fat effectively and mentally, rely on this nutritional form, you should give a fasting interval opportunity.

CHAPTER THREE

HOW TO START INTERMITTENT FASTING?

Intermittent fasting is psychologically more affordable for the "beginners of the fast" (less deprivation) and more comfortable implementing as a daily event in an ordinary social life. It can be done over a more extended period than complete fasting because it puts the organism (Body) less to the test. There is minimal risk of suffering a "healing crisis" (signs of detoxification such as migraines, digestive disorders, nausea, etc.) with intermittent fasting.

In practice, I recommend skipping dinner (or breakfast). It is simpler socially and less harsh for people who exercise a demanding professional activity. Only water (or herbal teas or broths) is allowed during the skipped meal. Start by doing this intermittent intermediate approach once a week (e.g., Sunday morning), then gradually increase until you find your cruising pace. This type of fasting can be done all through the year or over the space of a number of weeks.

Of course, to reap the benefits, for the rest of the day have a varied and balanced diet by limiting deli meats, red meat, dairy products, fries, pastries, and sweets! Choose Healthier options such as raw fruits and vegetables (whole or in juice, soups), whole grains and legumes, eggs, white meats, and fish!

All You Have to Know Before You Start

More and more people swear by interval fasting. While some want to get rid of annoying pounds, others want to promote their health by fasting. We'll tell you what the trends are and once you start fasting in this section, we will explain what you need to know. All right, read on...

No Normal Fasting Cure

Firstly, did you think that interval fasting, and intermittent fasting were one and the same? Well, read on. Intermittent fasting differs in some ways from other conventional fasting methods.

While with fasting practices such as Bachinger's fasting, the calorie intake is reduced over days or weeks, fasting during interval fasting often only by the hour.

Normal fasting is usually carried out once or twice a year. Intermittent fasting, on the other hand, is used daily or at least weekly.

Normal fasting cures are often used to detoxify the body. Such treatments are characterized by low-calorie intake and are often associated with a colon cleanse. This can be done either alone, at home, or in a clinic under medical supervision. These cures are supposed to free the so-called slags which build up within the digestive system and the associated suffering.

These methods are not suitable for losing weight.

Those who intermittently fast, on the other hand, have entirely different goals. Losing weight is often one of the main reasons because, with the interval, fasting pounds can disappear, without adversely affecting the metabolism, or diminishing muscle mass, in fact with regular Intermittent fasting, fat metabolism is positively influenced, the metabolism learns to use its reserves because the body breaks down fat and turns it into energy. This leads to weight loss without having to follow a strict diet.

Common Methods of Fasting

Interval fasting is the generic term for many methods, characterized by a regular Lent. While some ways only last for hours, others reduce their calorie intake for up to two days. Although, it should be noted that all methods should be part of everyday life, daily or weekly, to achieve a significant effect.

The 16: 8 method

The 16: 8 method is probably the best-known procedure for interval fasting. Here you fast for 16 hours a day and have a time window of 8 hours to eat meals. That means you miss a meal. This can either be breakfast or dinner. If you omit breakfast, you could eat in the time window from 12 noon to 8pm. If you prefer to miss dinner, there is a time slot from 9 a.m. to 5 p.m.

You can generally eat in the 8 hours when meals are taken. It works best if you do not restrict your calorie intake but also if you do not eat more than usual at those meals. Also, sugary and fatty foods are not forbidden, but a much better effect can be achieved and observed more quickly, if you have a balanced and healthy diet and It's good for your health too. You should not eat for four to five hours between meals. Snacks between the main meals can lead to food cravings and interrupt fat loss. It would be better to drink water or unsweetened herbal teas.

An example plan of Intermittent fasting with the 16: 8 method: and instructions:

- **7 a.m.:** Get up and drink plenty of water to kee[...] hydrated. Sports on an empty stomach can increas[...] consumption and boost metabolism. But it would be [...] you did not overdo it. Consider a short run or light train[...]

- **Morning:** Coffee is allowed during interval fasting. Fasting can, therefore, be bridged with a cup of black coffee. Tea is also available. However, drinks should be calorie-free. Sweetened beverages and latte coffee are out of the question.

- **Noon:** Fast breakage. The first meal is coming up. Since a meal is omitted daily, you should pay attention to sufficient calorie and nutritional intake. An active and healthy option is a wholesome meal with vegetables, egg whites, and whole grains. When eating, you should take your time and enjoy the meal.

- **Afternoon:** You should refrain from snacks here. But you can grab tea and coffee again. After16,00 however, it may be better abstaining from caffeine consumption so as not to impair the sleep rhythm.

- **19.00 (Last meal of the day):** Again, the best recommendation would be best if you went with a balanced meal. A dessert is also allowed but try to opt for a fruit salad or a quark-based dessert. You can drink a glass of wine or a beer for dinner, but alcohol should only be consumed in small quantities.

- **Evening:** At 20.00 begins the fasting. Now only water and caffeine-free teas should be consumed. Eight hours of sleep a night should provide adequate rest. So, in effect, you can sleep half the time of your fast and remember while you are sleeping your system is still working for your benefit.

The 5: 2 method

With this method, instead of fasting daily, your fasting is limited to two days a week. Five days a week, you can eat healthy meals and do not have to spend time fasting in between. Food intake is significantly reduced over the remaining two days. Women should consume only 500 calories per day and Men eat 600 calories a day, and as a result, carbohydrates are entirely dispensed. During these fasting periods, one should resort to vegetable broths, vegetables, and protein-containing foods. This method really works best if you always fast on the same days of the week or especially if you do it during the weekends as since the calorie intake is significantly reduced, you may be able to plan sufficient rest periods and less strenuous activities more easily.

Alternating fasting

Alternating fasting is made up of a typical day and a fasting day that always alternates. Another name for this method is "10 in 2". It stands for the one day you eat (1) and the fast day (0), which together make two days (2). Discipline is required here because the calorie intake is significantly reduced on the fasting day. While you do not have to pay attention to your diet for one day, you only eat vegetable broths, water, and unsweetened teas the following day. When feasting, you should not only resort to sugary and fatty foods. A balanced diet is essential so that the body receives all the necessary nutrients.

Alternatives: fast for 12 hours or one day a week

If these methods are too strict and you still want to try interval fasting, Shorten the fasting time slightly. Instead of fasting for 16 hours a day, you can start with 12 hours. Here, one sleeps most of the fasting period, in effect for eight hours with only four hours for a meal. A suitable time window would be, for example, a fast from 8 p.m.; to 8 a.m. So, you would have to do without dinner or breakfast.

If you prefer to fast every week instead of daily, you can start on a fasting day. Here you fast for 24 hours and feed exclusively on vegetable broths, water, teas, and juices. It would be best if you refrained from solid food. Fasting can be started either for breakfast, lunch, or dinner. There must be 24 consecutive hours.

Which is the best for women over 40?

Be aware of this:

Partial fasting affects the female hormone balance. Therefore, women over 40, in particular, should fast very carefully. It is quite possible that women may feel uncomfortable and fatigued during fasting.

Some perimenopausal women reported that when they are on the 16/8 diet, they:

- had no hot flashes at night.

- They are much more balanced emotionally.

- They have slept through the night.

- No longer had a racing heart or anxiety attacks at night.

If you are not sure whether intermittent fasting is suitable for you, you should consult your medical professional.

Note:

- Do not fast on consecutive days. Instead, fast, for example, Tuesday, Thursday, and Saturday.

- Do not fast for more than 12 to 13 hours. A fasting phase between 7 p.m. and 8 a.m. is ideal, for example. With a longer fasting window, a stress reaction is triggered.

- Do not train hard on fasting days. Instead of intense exercises like HIIT, long runs, or strength training, you should do yoga or a light cardio training set.

- Make sure you drink enough water when you fast.

- Your diet should be tailored to your hormonal needs and contain no inflammation triggering substances, such as gluten, sugar, dairy, or red meat.

- Particularly important: listen to your body. If you are not feeling well while fasting, have a headache, or are irritable, do not overdo it. Every woman is different and or bodies will react differently to fasting. Be careful with yourself and ensure that you take it easy on the days you fast.

CHAPTER FOUR

MYTHS ABOUT INTERMITTENT FASTING

When it comes to fasting, many myths continue to be disseminated even by health professionals. Here are five of those myths that you must stop believing when taking advantage of this nutritional approach's benefits.

Along with the ketogenic diet, fasting as a nutritional and dietary intervention has become popular recently. Practical and scientific reasons are not lacking. For many cases, a controlled fasting regime is better than simply adopting one of many popular restrictive diets. However, much information that we know today is wrong. It continues to be disseminated even by health professionals who do not get rid of conceptions promoted for decades, becoming nutritional dogma. For example, we need to eat three times a day. But here we have, backed by serious scientific studies, most carried out in recent decades, five of the most widespread myths wrong about fasting, a style of food that is neither new nor dangerous.

And if it is a fad, why has it been around for hundreds of thousands of years.

1. Skipping breakfast makes you fat

This myth continues to spread, as done by nutritionists. The idea that breakfast is the most important meal of the day is only true when the daily diet is (badly) based on carbohydrates.

Studies have already shown that overweight and obese people showed no difference in weight in 16 weeks, whether they ate breakfast or not. Other studies suggest that the opposite is true: those who lose weight in the long term eat breakfast often. What you eat and when you eat the rest of the day's meals influences your metabolism, but in general, it is a good practice not to have breakfast until you starve yourself.

Also, skipping breakfast will only make you fat if what you eat later will be foods high in calories and low in healthy fats, protein, and micronutrients, such as flours, pasta, and sugars.

So, don't blame the fact of not having breakfast, but instead blame the poor nutritional quality of what you eat when you do eat if you have skipped breakfast.

2. Regular eating improves your metabolism, reduces appetite, helps you lose weight, and is good for your health

As we can see by the increase in obesity, diabetes, and all other Metabolic Syndrome members in recent decades, eating three or more times a day is not the solution to achieve a healthy weight.

Contrary to what the traditional professional council says, we do not need to eat three times a day. This advice comes from a custom that has only existed since the industrial revolution when working hours made it necessary to establish food schedules.

Recent studies proved that regular eating promotes the storage of calories in the form of fat, which over time encourages diabetes and many other chronic conditions related to excess calories. In other words, eating more times a day does not increase the metabolic rate nor reduce hunger, much less help you lose weight; however, it does affect the nutrient composition of what you eat and how your body is able to manage these calories metabolically.

3. Your brain needs a regular intake of food glucose

Yet another great myth that is a product of the food industry's approach in the last 100 years and not a fact-based on the human body's metabolic functioning.

To date, the nutritional standard continues to consider the consumption of carbohydrates in the composition of food necessary because "carbohydrates provide energy." And yes, while they do provide energy, that energy is useful only in the short term. Carbohydrates are cheap fuel and easy to burn, but also far too easy to store. And it is not essential.

The human body can easily produce more and better energy from fats. Also, human metabolism evolved to synthesize the glucose necessary for the brain and other tissues of other macronutrients such as lipids and proteins. So, we do not need carbohydrates from food directly. And much less refined carbohydrates.

We now know what the Inuit and all our ancestors took advantage of: the human body, including the brain, works best in a state of ketosis, that is, with fat as its primary source of energy and no carbohydrates.

4. Fasting puts your body in starvation mode and makes you lose muscle

As we discussed in an earlier chapter, it is an urban legend that muscle is lost only by fasting. As we also summarize, combining exercise and fasting is better for many reasons.

However, we do not stop listening to the advice of eating before exercising that fasting encourages the famous state of starvation. According to this myth, if we don't eat for several hours or days, our body will eat itself, and the muscle will degrade when the opposite is what happens.

We now know from various studies that the state of fasting encourages hormones that promote muscle preservation and development. If this myth of the "starvation mode" were true, the human race would have long since died out in one of many seasons of food shortages. As Dr. Jason Fung explains in many of his talks on the subject, "the body is not stupid" and is evolved to consume muscle proteins only as a last resort, precisely because muscle is what it takes to move in search of food.

5. Fasting makes you overeat

Clear. But only when it is your habit to feed yourself with meals of little nutritional value. When what we eat are calories that are saved or burned quickly, we will eat much more than necessary if we wait several hours to eat. However, as in the case of preserved and even gained muscle, fasting by eating the right foods will help you need less food to function the same and better. Once the adaptation time has passed (which differs depending on your eating and genetic habits), fasting for a longer time will be easier, and not vice versa, as many people, including health professionals, still believe.

It's that simple: several studies have already proven that fasting reduces insulin levels, increases metabolic rate (the rate at which you burn calories), norepinephrine, and growth hormone levels; what makes you lose fat, not gain it. And that is why intermittent fasting is becoming famous as an intervention to lose weight and combat conditions such as diabetes.

How to Take Advantage of The Benefits of Fasting?

Fasting, as we have seen in the explanations for all of these myths, has many benefits for metabolism and health in general, among them and very importantly, is the activation of what is considered a system of self-protection of the body that evolved originally to ensure the survival of our species; but now we can take advantage to live longer and with greater health.

But this is the subject of some of the following chapters, on intermittent fasting, the most practical technique to integrate fasting into our diet and to take advantage of all the benefits of emulating the way our ancestors fed for hundreds of thousands of years.

CHAPTER FIVE

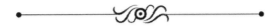

WHEN SHOULD YOU AVOID INTERMITTENT FASTING?

Intermittent fasting has proven to be an effective and interesting method to help in the fight against overweight. However, it is not always convenient to get carried away by this nutritional pattern's fame. And, in some cases, intermittent fasting could prove harmful. What cases are we talking about?

As we have mentioned at several points already, intermittent fasting is an interesting and effective method of promoting fat consumption and weight loss. Of course, it is no miracle system, and its effects may not be noticed immediately. However, evidence has shown that this system has long-term benefits.

Fasting for 12 to 20 hours in a row, can, lower risk factors for cardiovascular and metabolic disorders and even reverse some of their effects. Practitioners of this pattern have also been shown to have a reduced chance of cancer and neurodegenerative disorders. While we don't know at this point what exact processes are involved in this, they are most likely based on our circadian rhythms.

What are Circadian Rhythms?

Circadian rhythms are physical, mental, and behavioral changes that follow a 24-hour cycle. These natural processes respond primarily to light and dark and affect most living things, including animals, plants, and microbes. Chronobiology is the study of circadian rhythms.

They control the metabolism by segregating melatonin and a cascade of signals that stimulate our body. If we consider it from the evolutionary perspective, the circadian rhythm has been adapted through thousands of years of evolution to fasting. But before embarking on practicing it, we must bear in mind that there are some people who at all costs should not practice intermittent fasting.

When Should Intermittent Fasting Not Be Practiced?

It must be noted that intermittent fasting (and fasting in general) has not shown any problem or harm outside of these cases. Moreover, it has been shown to have an important series of benefits: blood glucose level control, cardiovascular problem control, cancer prevention. However, it is better to take care of yourself in the following cases:

When you need a lot of energy

Not all bodies work the same, nor do all bodies need the same amount of energy. If we need a large number of calories, intermittent fasting is completely contraindicated. What occasions do we mean? Normally in the case of being underweight (with a BMI below 18.5).

The is especially important because the body is a machine to consume energy, and it is also contraindicated when in a growing phase, for example if, someone under the age of 18 decides that they want to perform this dietary pattern; you must first consult a doctor or a professional dietitian-nutritionist.

Also, it is also totally out of place when there is an eating disorder, such as anorexia or bulimia.

When we suffer from sleep problems

Intermittent fasting, especially when you start the practice, can change many of our habits, that includes our sleep, which can be affected in a very unpleasant way. The change of pattern has important metabolic consequences.

If an individual suffers from insomnia or similar problems, we should avoid intermittent fasting. In short, the issues that will arise from not sleeping will not be compensated by the benefits of the fast.

When there are anxiety problems such as stress

As with sleep, if an individual suffers from stress or anxiety, it is better to leave intermittent fasting aside. Changing our metabolic pattern can be costly at the mood level, and our mood will suffer a lot.

Again, the fault lies with our metabolism, which increases hormones that signal alertness and make us more aggressive and predisposed to depression.

In addition, anxious behaviors can translate into something else: compulsive eating. This happens many more often than you may think. As we have said other times, the period of intake of intermittent fasting is not equal to a white letter from the binge, in which we can eat everything we want and how much we want. In cases such as this food must follow a healthy and adequate pattern and in these types of cases (as in any other), compulsive eating goes against the ultimate goal, and in effect "the remedy can be worse than the disease. "

When there are metabolic problems

In high uric acid production problems, metabolic syndrome, or even diabetes, intermittent fasting is discouraged. It is not that it cannot be practiced, but, at the very least, we should consult with a specialist medical professional, who can tell us what we can and cannot do and how we should do it. This way we will avoid serious problems and unpleasant surprises that could end very badly.

These reasons are due to the metabolic change that drives intermittent fasting. Used to living in a constant intake cycle, all metabolisms will be pressured to change our blood glucose levels, fat mobilization, changes in the cascade of hormones and signals. In this very complex process, we could jeopardize some important steps for our health. If we suffer from a disease, it is best to be well informed by a specialist medical practitioner, before embarking on the adventure of fasting.

CHAPTER SIX

HOW CAN I LOSE SOME WEIGHT IN A MONTH?

Let's figure out what would be necessary to achieve this. If we believe we will lose about 5lbs every ten days for 30 days per month (Approximately 2 kg or 15 lb. in 3 days or 0.5 lb./day or more than 3lbs per week).

As example's I will take an imaginary man and woman and put down some figures for them. From these examples you'll be able to work out for yourself how to do it if you're different from these examples. If we conclude that there are about 3500 calories are in a pound of fat and want to get those 3lbs off (3500 x 3lbs = Cals), you need to build a deficit of at least 10500 calories every week. That works out to a daily deficit of about 1,500 calories if we break that down into everyday loss.

Now, let's find out how much energy a body needs:

Here are some examples, let's take three men and three women.

Male 1

- 70kg -11st 3lb - 154.3lbs

- Cals (range) of energy 1,918-3,036

Male 2

- 80 kg — 12st 4 lb. — 176.4lbs

- Cals (range) of energy 2.038-3.226.

Male 3

- 90 kg-14st 4 lb-198.4lbs

- Cals (range) of energy 2,158-3,416 Cals.

Female 1

- 60 kg — 9st 3 lb. — 132.3lbs

- Cals (range) of energy 1,598-2,531

Female 2

- 70kg -11st 3lb - 154.3lbs

- Cals (range) of energy-1,718-2,721

Female 3

- 80 kg-12st 4 lb-176.4lbs

- Cals (range) of energy 1,838-2,911 Cals

Notes:

The ranges for daily calorie expenditure can vary considerably depending on the individual activity level, from a sedentary lifestyle (for instance, an office worker who drives to work and takes no or extremely limited exercise) to a highly active lifestyle (someone with a job involving several hours of manual work per day or exercises at a high intensity with a consistently high heart rate per day for more than 90 minutes.

These fictional figures are based on someone in their mid-30s, who is about 170 cm tall, and they are used for illustration purposes only; the principles behind the practices here are valid; but you will obviously need to personalize your situation. These are averages only and will vary from person to person; you need to get your starting figures to find out more accurately. You can use the calculators found on a variety of different apps or websites to do this. For a rough starting point, use the BMR (Basal metabolic rate) and RMR (resting energy expenditure – which is the number of calories your body burns while it's at rest) calculations, then use the techniques to change the figures based on the real world's results for a 60 kg woman, who is only mildly active or passive!

So, in that scenario, you can see that this would mean no eating at all for about a month. That outcome would definitely not work for us! What it is important to note is that a 60 kg woman doesn't have to lose 14lbs (about 6 kg) or more than 10% of her body weight, so we don't have to worry about those results. The upper end of the scale is what we should be looking. That is where the large numbers in respect of weight loss are very realistic.

For example, if you look at the 90 kg man, even a passive person could cut off more than 1000 calories from their daily intake, as long as they do it with the right foods. In a little, I'm going to come to that. Firstly, let's look briefly at the three factors that will allow for this significant calorie reduction..................................

1: Intermittent Fasting

Intermittent fasting (the version of Lean gains 16/8) is a simple way to feed the body. You divide the day into two phases, a phase of eating and a phase of not eating. It takes about 8 hours to eat. The fasting period thus lasts roughly 16 hours. **This does not mean you're eating the whole 8-hour block!**

There are two key aspects to Intermittent Fasting that make massive weight loss work for you.

One, physiologically, is that every day is divided into two distinct phases, each of which helps your fat loss goal. These two phases are an anabolic or tissue-building phase and a fat-burning or energy breakdown phase.

Two, using "IF" makes it much easier than traditional diets to reduce your calories: You should definitely try "IF" if you want to make your weight loss as painless and effective as possible.

2: Food high Protein, low-fat, low carbon

In his excellent series of posts on developing a diet for fat loss, Lyle MacDonald talks about setting it up from the ground instead of from the top. What are we saying? Okay, what we've done here is to start with a target of weight loss, which is the top or limit, and then work backward to determine what we need to do. Lyle takes a slightly different approach in those papers, works out what you need physiologically, and then brings those figures into a diet to see what ends up coming out. Here we will use part of that strategy (setting protein intake) to give you a starting point for finding out what you are eating.

How Much Food Do You Need?

Looking things more precisely, how much protein in each meal will you strive for? Well, we can answer this question in two ways; the best answer is the one that makes you feel most reassured. The quick answer is 'lots.' The more precise response is worked out as follows; begin with a bodyweight level of about 1g / lb. of body weight and break it down over your two or three meals, then change based on lean tissue and decrease in strength and levels of hunger/satiety. So, if you find your strength falling and your muscle leaving your body, you need to add more protein to it, and if you feel hungry between meals or are not happy with a meal, add more protein!

What Foods Can I Eat?

I consistently find that this type of fasting regime, does not increase the appetite and that there are no feelings of deprivation, which should not be shocking given the enormous range of foods on offer here. You will notice the total lack of powders/protein drinks for liquid foods/meal substitution. This is deliberate; they do not provide satiety and fulfillment, and they provide no incentive. "Don't drink your calories," as Martin Berkhan says.

Why High Protein, Low Fat, Low Carb?

A few reasons.

1. **, you want the calories to be kept as low as possible, as easily as possible**.

2. **, protein plus lots of bulky yet low-carbon foods**

These make it easy to feel full, satisfied, and happy when you cut calories.

3. **: Doing only high-intensity weights and very low-intensity cardio**

Each of the three elements is equally important in this weight loss plan, so you'd better find a way of including this part! Just ask yourself if it's worth jeopardizing the whole plan for the sake of missing some simple exercises.

Why start with a statement like that?

Since slipping back into old ways of intensely training for weight loss is just way too easy for many people, what you need to do is heavy weights with low reps and using as big as possible movements. Remember, large weights are totally specific to each individual. The actual number/weight is irrelevant; what is important is that you lift to YOUR ability and learn how to lift fully at your ability.

This means learning what a max effort lift feels like AND expecting the max to go up quickly while you know how to get more and more out of yourself for those of you who have hardly lifted weights before.

Remember to check with your Healthcare professional before embarking on a training program.

The great thing about this program is that it is easy. Take and repeat the following exercises:

- Squat
- Dumbbell press, bench press, or bodyweight dips
- Dumbbell or barbell shoulder press
- Lat pull-down, pull-up, sitting row, or bent over Deadlift barbell/dumbbell
- track.

Your rotation is easy: Do five sets of 4-6 reps for three weeks (routine 5x5 style) and then three weeks of 9-12 reps (routine 3x10 style). You increase the weight every time you hit the upper rep range. You only have to rest after 10-14 weeks (but if you've regularly been training for more than twelve weeks, you need to take a week of complete rest right now-unless you're planning within 12 weeks from the beginning of your plan, in which case you'll get your rest at the end!)

Suppose you don't know how these exercises can be done. In that case, you should take instructions from a competent trainer (you can find out if they're good by watching how they get you to move and focus on your learning exercises, if they get you to do your exercises like those done in instruction videos, you can be sure they know their stuff), or you can check out the abundance of videos on YouTube and figure it out using those.

CHAPTER SEVEN

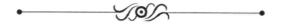

HOW THE WOMAN'S BODY CHANGES

Or body does not stop changing throughout our lives. Age and genetics are primarily responsible for these changes, although they are not the only factors. External factors such as tobacco, alcohol, poor diet, or excessive sunbathing are also determinant factors for our health's deterioration over the decades.

In women's case, the number of hormones that they have determines our bodies' evolution over the decades. Fertility is also key to understanding the changes that occur. "Between the decades of the 20s and 60s, the woman body undergoes a series of important changes, both hormonally and physically, as a result of menstrual cycles, pregnancies, and other derivatives of reproductive aging.

At 20 years old

During this decade, the woman is full of energy and performance, and we enjoy a baseline health status. The body adapts to our rhythm of life, and we perform better physically.

Genetics are a fundamental factor that determines endogenous aging. However, everything takes its toll. As much as at 20 years, the skin is full of collagen, a weekend of excesses on the beach or smoking are points that accumulate against the epidermis and time. "If a person with a genetic predisposition to have a thinner dermis or lighter skin, also smokes, sunbathes, and practices excessive facial gesture's, they may end up having wrinkles in their 20s.

Creating good eating and exercise habits while avoiding alcohol and smoking and paying attention to eating disorders, as well as attending gynecological exams every year can go a long way.

As for the skin, during this decade and the third, the woman loses the brightness of adolescence and therefore must start using moisturizers, which should preferably be rich in alpha-hydroxy acids.

During the second decade, the woman is in the fullness of her sexual development in respect of ovarian activity. The secretion of hormones such as estrogen and progesterone play a fundamental role in the menstrual cycle and fertility.

At birth, a woman's ovaries have a million oocytes and will no longer produce after that. In each menstrual cycle, they are discarded, so as time progresses, the possibility of becoming a mother decreases until menopause arrives. Between the ages of 15 and 25, the probability of becoming pregnant in each cycle is 40 percent. During this time, contraceptive treatments should be considered in order to avoid unwanted pregnancy and reduce the transmission of infectious diseases.

At age 30

From the age of 30, there begins to be a decrease in metabolism, which means that we naturally burn fewer calories per minute if we do not exercise. The specialist Concepción de Lucas points out that your physical condition can worsen with work stress or poor diet and also if you also lead a sedentary lifestyle.

Also, this is the decade in which many women choose to have their first child. Some experts point out that this moment is key for women. "In this decade, muscle tone can easily be lost, and, with pregnancy, the body can undergo significant changes, with increases and decreases in weight, body volume, and muscle sagging."

It is also common to observe adult acne, which usually appears in the jaw area, and that is due to excessive sensitivity of the skin in that area due to hormonal changes. It can often be treated with oral contraceptive treatments or oral recurrences (not indicated for pregnant women since it can cause alterations in the fetus) or topological applications and as dermatologist María Teresa Truchuelo explains. This type of acne may also be due to disorders such as the polycystic ovary syndrome or the use of overly fatty cosmetics.

From the age of 30, expression wrinkles may begin to appear in the areas where we are most gesturing, such as between the eyebrows or the eye area, with bags and crow's feet. The dermatology specialists recommend using moisturizers containing active ingredients such as the alpha hydroxy acids, which seek to reshape the skin or vitamin C, and niacinamide.

During this decade it is really important to maintain good eating and exercise habits, go to gynecological exams annually and do health checks to monitor cholesterol, weight, visual and auditory understanding, and the early detection of diseases and pathologies.

From the age of 35, the woman's fertility starts to noticeably decrease. It can be increasingly difficult to get pregnant, so gynecologists advise not to delay motherhood beyond this age. In addition to having to resort to assisted reproduction techniques, it can also add the risks of having a miscarriage, hypertension,

31

diabetes, and deformations or alterations in the fetus. From the age of 35- 40, the probability of pregnancy in each cycle is drops to 25 percent.

At age 40

During the fourth decade of our life, a huge series of changes in our physiognomy begin to become quite apparent. The fat that had occurred predominantly in the buttocks and legs previously for reproductive purposes, now, begins to redistribute itself in the abdomen, increasing the risk of cardiovascular disease. It also, results in significant decreases in both muscle tone and mass and increases begin in the start of sagging in certain areas of the arms and legs, especially if we do not exercise.

The level of hormones in our bodies also drops significantly during this decade and as this is most usually when a woman is moving away from her period of fertility. Skin noticeably starts to show loss of elasticity, and sunspots begin to develop like antigens, which do tend to be more marked on lighter skins. "Expression wrinkles intensify, and facial volumes begin to vary. It is generally at this point that the Dermatology expert recommends anti-spot lasers, botulinum toxin for expression wrinkles, and hyaluronic acid to treat the nasogenial grooves, wrinkles and volume loss.

This is where good eating habits, good nutrition and exercise start to become really important, and these will contribute to a better preparation for menopausal transition.

Also, it is around this time that along with obvious external signs of significant change appearing externally that the intervertebral discs can begin to become compressed, and it is normal for spine pain and loss of muscle tone to increase, and even osteoporosis or loss of bone mass to begin to occur.

However, that having been said, there is still a lot that young women can to do slow the onset of the appearance of these things, by adopting a diet rich in calcium and performing muscle strength exercises. These serve to condition the muscles and make them as strong as possible. They also strengthen the union of muscle to bone via the tendons.

From the ages of 40 - 50 years old, women can begin to notice hot flashes, irritability, difficulty sleeping, vaginal dryness, decreased libido, and alterations in menstruation; At this point, "We are premenopausal," explains Esparza, who advises seeing it as "a natural stage in women," which must be normalized and treated if necessary, to reduce any symptoms. "We must not fear it or feel there are methods to prevent it, accept it as another this stage both in our development as a person and as a woman".

It is usually accepted that menopause occurs most often between the ages of 45 and 55 years old, however recent studies have shown much more frequency in the occurrence of early menopause onsets, often in women in their late 30's or early 40's and there are a number of research studies that are looking into the reasons behind this.

From 50 years old

During their 50s, most women begin to suffer from menopause, which is the absence of menstruation for more than 12 months and is due to the permanent cessation of follicular function. Its diagnosis is clinical and retrospective when 12 months have elapsed since the last period without any menstrual bleeding.

There are no "absolute" guidelines on how to deal with the Menopause, because each woman is different and will have a different experience, but most of the changes in their bodies around this age are directly related to it." Some women sail through

Menopause with no discernable symptoms, although that tends to be the exception rather than the rule. Most women will have some symptoms and others will experience all of them.

During this period, the alteration in the distribution of body fat continues. The skin's appearance in terms of elasticity and hydration worsens, vaginal dryness and other mucous membranes that can cause pain during sexual intercourse may be experienced, muscle tone decreases, and muscle mass deteriorates. Often Osteoarthritis problems appear together with problems of the spine, joints, or bones.

"It also increases cardiovascular risk, sleep and memory disorders may also be influenced by the gradual loss of estrogen," explain some specialists, adding that lifestyle changes can also cause several mood changes: "during this stage. It is also normal to suffer more anxiety, depression and a decrease in or marked variances in mood."

In the fifth decade, the woman may also notice that she loses pubic and auxiliary hair, undergoes changes in hair and skin, or increases body weight. Menopause causes considerable changes between 50 and 60 years and a woman's skin experience may undergo many alterations. "The not insignificant decrease in estrogen that occurs around this time in the woman's life leads to a thinning of the skin and marked signs of dehydration, which causes wrinkles to intensify and 'sagging' of structures.

The body can be acclimatized to the symptoms of menopause by reducing body temperature by wearing light clothing, drinking plenty of cold drinks, especially water and by exercising regularly to prevent osteoporosis. Optimizing nutrition, doing controlled breathing exercises, and going to gynecological exams and other medical check-ups are also tips to keep in mind during this stage and during the sixth decade of our life.

Specialists agree that "throughout a woman's life, the gynecologist must be present, adapting her actions to her different health and reproductive status". At every ageing stage of the woman, physical changes and psychological changes occur, and specialists should be able to provide advice at any or all these stages. These are vital phases that must be accepted and lived. Every change you do not understand or doubt that you have, it is wise to consult your gynecologist as it is more than likely that they will be able to provide useful information and have answers for you.

Implementation of Physical Activity

Incorporating moderate physical activity into a daily routine induces a series of physiological changes in the body that go beyond burning calories, reducing fat, and maintaining muscle mass. In addition to promoting weight loss and improving the relationship between food and the body itself, physical activity induces a change in the body's composition and the functioning of metabolism and systems (circulatory, respiratory, etc.). Daily physical exercise, for example, is a way to improve cardiovascular health because it acts on different fronts:

- It reduces blood pressure, favoring the control of hypertension.

- Increases the secretion of HDL cholesterol (good cholesterol), reducing the rate of blood cholesterol.

- It induces a decrease in triglyceride levels.

It decreases insulin production, helping to control type 2 diabetes, favoring the assimilation of nutrients and their arrival in the cells of the different cell tissues, and reducing fat uptake and accumulation.

Physical activity

Control of cardiovascular risk factors (hypercholesterolemia, arterial hypertension, and type 2 diabetes).

- It increased lung capacity.

- Increase in muscle strength and mass.

- Increase in aerobic capacity.

- Reduction of fat mass.

- It improves the person's psychological balance by inducing personal satisfaction and the control of anxiety and stress.

Finally, it is worth highlighting one last benefit of physical activity; it improves the individual's relationship with food, reduces appetite, and favors adopting healthy eating habits.

Conditions of Use of the Service

In no way can the information provided by this tool replace a direct health care provider, nor should it be used to determine a diagnosis or choose a procedure in particular cases.

No recommendation on drugs, techniques, products, etc., will be made in this information, explicitly or implicitly. This can only be viewed as a source of knowledge. The users are entirely responsible for their actions while using this program. The details you see in these examples are those which can be found in any fitness book or diet book and are no substitute for advice from your medical practitioner. With whom you should always check before embarking on any kind of diet or exercise program.

What Are the Types of Exercises That Are the Best for You (A Woman Over 40)?

It is time to set the table, You can join a gym or buy a cd or watch a YouTube video to find a vast amount of exercise options that you can use to exercise with and below are some easy basic exercises that may also be followed, However, it is always wise to consult your health care provider or your gym coach to ensure that any exercises that you do are appropriate for your specific needs.

It is widely accepted that any exercises from the age of 40 onwards should be aimed at achieving a fit and healthy body; the following exercises work a number of muscles in your body, including the buttocks and hamstrings which is important for women over 40, to create stronger, thinner legs that have enough force, to lift its rear part, with the quadriceps also working and don't forget to to ensure that the knees be strengthened with resistance work.

To perform the first of these exercises, stand in front of a bench or a firm chair, place your left foot firmly on top of the bench or chair, press your left foot and push the body back until the left leg is straight, lower the body down until the right knee is flexed and repeat 10 to 15 times. Weight balanced evenly, don't lean too far forward or too far back. The so-called bridge exercises are not only the perfect exercise for a perfectly rounded back, but they will also help women keep their back healthy and pain-free.

Define Abs for Women

To do a bridge, lay down on the floor neck and back relaxed, legs slightly bent. Feet flat on the floor, lift your hips so that your body curves, take a curved path from the shoulders to the knees, stop in the upper position for two or three seconds, and lower your body down to the original position; repeat 10 to 15 times.

Routine Abdominals for Women

The addition of raising an arm while performing the previous exercise on the floor improves the posture and the strength of the base, making you feel better. It will seem more effortless, but you will feel more secure. Given the aim of reducing our belly, it is important to perform the exercises consistently and linearly. It is advisable to expand the abdominal table for women progressively; every 10 or 15 days would be correct because each time, we will have further strengthened the abdominal area.

Strengthen Buttocks

To perform the following exercise for women over 40 to create stronger legs and buttocks, start by adopting an iron position, but bend your elbows and lean on your forearms instead of on your hands.

Exercise Table for The Buttocks

Your body should create a straight line to the ankles from the shoulders, tighten your buttocks and maintain your hip position while raising your right arm forward, move your shoulder blades down and back as you raise your arms, keep the position for 5 to 10 seconds relax the buttocks and repeat the exercise ten to fifteen times changing arm.

There are many physical and mental advantages of yoga, from investment postures that are excellent for helping to minimize the presence of cellulite, shoulder support, or raising the legs above the wall for 5 minutes a night before bed, which would be helpful not just for the appearance of cellulite but also for significantly aiding with its circulation.

Exercises for Women Over 40 Years to Create Thinner, And Stronger Legs.

To correctly perform the following exercise especially after the age of 40, you have to take this exercise more calmly and not rush it. To create stronger, more firm legs and buttocks, lie on your back and gradually lift your hips and legs off the floor, bringing your legs above your head until your toes touch the ground behind you, place your hands behind your back and extend your legs stretching them in the air, creating a straight line from your shoulders to your ankles.

Keep your neck relaxed and your shoulders supported; try to hold the position for at least one minute and then slowly return to the starting position, pause, rest, and then repeat the movement about ten more times, obviously using your respective breaks.

For quicker results in toning of the whole body, go through the movements described above and perform three sets of these exercises about ten times each or as otherwise indicated by a medical condition; transition at a steady pace between the movements, but don't rush the movements themselves.

The following day try to do other exercises, you can alternate between a couple of programs to give some variety and slowly begin to incorporate a few series of cardio intervals at the time of training your entire body, or you can do it separately over a longer period in these exercises for women over 40 years of age.

Choose workouts that work on certain areas and integrate them into the everyday routine to strengthen a particular area. Just note that to keep pushing the body and as you progress you will need to begin to raise the number of repetitions in the proportion that gets better results.

Some specialized exercises for Women Over 40

Multidirectional exercises help immensely to develop coordination and control while providing toning and hardening of the quadriceps, buttocks, hamstrings, and inner thighs.

These Exercises after 40 will help keep your back healthy and pain-free.

To make a move, stand with your feet aligned, both arms extended above your shoulders, palms facing upward, take a lunge move on your right foot diagonally into the corner of the space at a 45-degree angle, bending the right knee and touching the lower part of your body in a forward motion on your right hip, the back leg should be level, with your heel raised off the floor then alternate, start with 5 times on each side, progressively increasing.

Leg and buttock exercises

If you can touch the ground, do it on both sides of your right foot, lightly with your fingers, push with your right foot to return to the starting position, repeat 15 times on one leg and 15 times for the other, an option to modify this exercise is not to go so low in the stride and aim to reach with your hands at the knee or the level of the chin instead.

Leg exercises for women

Stand with your feet Hip width apart and focus on working out the abdominals with tight buttocks, squeezing your thighs together, and maintaining good posture.

In addition to getting thinner and stronger legs, these are postures that we must adapt to maintain a healthy and erect back. In addition to toning our legs, it will help our posture on a day-to-day basis and will help us to have a better quality of life.

CHAPTER EIGHT

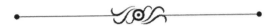

HOW TO USE PSYCHOLOGY TO PURSUE THE REGIME CONSTANTLY AND IN THE RIGHT WAY

What we eat affects how we feel, and how we feel impacts how we eat. As a result, there is a division of psychology devoted to looking after our eating patterns. It's generally referred to as diet psychology or food psychology.

Psychology and food are a match made in heaven for our well-being. While many people do not accept it, psychology may help people adhere to their diets by increasing body trust or controlling unhealthy food intake in obese people. There are psychological influences related to diet efficiency.

As a result, counselors are specialists who can help individuals improve their habits or their lifestyles. A successful dietary schedule can be carried out using tools (such as proper preparation, stimulus avoidance, and so on).

A counselor can be particularly useful in the battle against obesity, as emotional factors play a major role in achieving long-term improvements in eating habits. Also, in serious eating disorders, a psychologist is an important figure in the proper treatment of pathologies.

Eating with the eyes and tastes is a pleasant behavior.

Many individuals do not eat in compliance with their dietary criteria, but their eyes and tastes, drive them to ingest food without restriction. This can seem to be 'a routine practice, but it may be highly detrimental to one's health if foods of poor nutritional value and high amounts of harmful substances (such as trans fats) are eaten.

Abusing the pleasurable act of feeding will not only leave us sleepy and make us want to eat more, but it can also lead to severe health issues. Eating with the eyes and tastes is a pleasurable task, and consequently, the reward system, regulated by dopamine, is enabled. Dopamine is a neurotransmitter that tends to promote pleasurable habits like sex and substance use.

Emotions Affect Our Diet: Emotional Eating

People also have a strong idea of food pedagogy; the issue is that they do not adopt an eating schedule for several reasons, including a lack of inspiration, ambitious expectations, pessimistic self-efficacy values, sensitivity to interfering factors, and a poor mood.

We are more likely to eat fatty foods during periods of emotional instability, so the connection between emotions and diet is evident. This is bad for weight loss which induces an accumulation of fat in the diet. Emotional eating is where we use food to help us deal with our feelings.

Social and emotional considerations are crucial for the diet's progress because it is not easy for many people. On the other hand, we must understand individual nature and acknowledge that certain people consume a lot of food in response to anxiety or emotional problems. Stress also impacts mood, which affects food consumption.

Depression and Binge Eating

Depressed people sometimes increase their food intake disproportionately in serious conditions such as depression. Periods of overeating can occur during the depression but without loss of control (something that does occur in binge eating disorder).

Many foods contain tryptophan, an amino acid that activates serotonin development, which is why people suffering from stress or mental disease often turn to diet to make them feel better and relax (low levels of serotonin are associated with depression and obsession).

Fear, depression, and irritability are only a couple of the harmful consequences of a lack of serotonin in the body. Since the body does not produce tryptophan, it must be ingested by the diet. As a consequence, foods abundant in this amino acid have antidepressant properties.

Serotonin has been related to a greater sense of well-being, happiness, better sleep, higher self-esteem, better focus, and a better mood in many studies. Serotonin plays a vital part in the brain since it controls other neurotransmitters' balance, including dopamine and norepinephrine. These neurotransmitters are important because they are linked to anxiety, anxiety disorders, and eating disorders.

Foods to Improve Our Well-Being

This is the list of foods rich in tryptophan:

- Turkey

- Chicken

- Milk

- Cheese

- Fish

- Eggs

- Tofu

- Soy

- Walnuts

- Chocolate

- Chia seeds

Finally, low amounts of the neurotransmitter serotonin have been related to obsessive habits and binge eating disorder. Estrogen can improve serotonin production, which may help to avoid binge eating.

Psychology Applied to Nutrition

There is a connection between psychology and diet, as we previously mentioned. The field of "Nutrition Psychology" is concerned with studying and applying these processes in normal and abnormal contexts. For a person's healthy growth, the connection between psychism, social, mental, educational influences, and diet is crucial.

We have been taught to absorb the beauty in the Western world due to the current socio-economic structure. If the consequences of body culture are not reduced, pathologies or eating behavior problems such as Anorexia or Bulimia evolve. The importance of psychology on individuals' safe growth is important because of the need for collaboration between diet and mental health disciplines.

Obesity, for example, isn't just about gaining weight; in many situations, there are other causes at stake that must be tackled as well. A person who has been obese since childhood has never had his slender body portrayed. The changes you make would have an effect not just on your weight but also on your identity. Consequently, psychology plays an important role in people's well-being, and diet is an important part of a person's overall development.

CHAPTER NINE

CLEANING SYSTEM WITH AUTOPHAGY

Autophagy is the body's way of cleaning out damaged cells, in order to regenerate newer, healthier cells, "Auto" means self, and "phage" means eat. So, the literal meaning of **autophagy** is "self-eating."

Damaged cells and those that have developed to their critical limit, if they accumulate, can trigger inflammatory pathways that damage our health and lead to the emergence of diseases, including neurodegenerative diseases such as Parkinson's or Alzheimer's.

Cells degrade and reuse their unusable components through this phase of autophagy. This is used to obtain energy and reuses smaller molecules using them as cell renewal bricks. They are also responsible for destroying and removing the remains of bacteria and viruses after infection, eliminating damaged proteins, and counteracting aging's negative effects.

This mechanism has long been known, discovered in the sixties. In 2016, the scientific community awarded Dr. Yoshinori Ohsumi the Nobel Prize in medicine for his discoveries in this field. Researchers recognize autophagy as a survival system through which the body protects itself.

Is Autophagy Excellent or is it Bad for Us?

While the word's etymology gives a meaning that repels (the term eating yourself just doesn't sound right), it is a natural cellular renewal mechanism. This plays a key role in the prevention of autoimmune, neurodegenerative and indeed infectious diseases.

Furthermore, as it removes and reuses damaged parts, it has anti-aging benefits. Inside the vacuoles, this process is carried out and some of the resulting products are reused again.

Benefits of Autophagy

The benefits at the cellular level of this process are being investigated. Some of the most important are:

- It provides cell energy and structure-forming elements.

- Recycles the remains of degraded protein and unusable parts of the cell.

- It has beneficial effects on heart cells and protects against heart disease.

- Removes damaged endoplasmic structures

- It protects DNA integrity.

- The nervous system is covered, and its cells are strengthened. Autophagy seems to improve the structure of the brain, cognitive function, and neuroplasticity.

- By removing intracellular pathogens, it increases immune function.

- It regulates the functions of mitochondria.

- It prevents necrosis of tissue.

Connection Between the Mechanisms of Autophagy and Cell Death

Apoptosis is the cell death mechanism that is part of an organism's normal development cycle. Many researchers believe that in removing ribosomes and protein aggregates, autophagy is selective. Several experiments have shown that an autophagic process is independent of apoptosis as a form of cell death.

These processes are remarkably interesting for scientists because it is believed that autophagy can help treat cancer and neurodegenerative diseases. This mechanism would protect those cells that we don't want to die and destroy the harmful ones.

How Can Autophagy Be Induced?

This mechanism is involved in all cells but increases in nutrient deficiency situations. It means that we can use stimuli such as intense exercise or fasting to activate this cycle.

Studies are ongoing to demonstrate that increasing autophagy favors weight loss or age-related disease control. But how can autophagy be induced?

Practice fasting

This is a quite a simple concept. It is about restricting food intake for a specific period. You can drink water or coffee, but you should not introduce any caloric food into the body. It is typically done following a strategy called intermittent fasting that limits the number of hours a day you eat, 4 or 8 as per your schedule. You don't eat anything the rest of the time.

Take for example, breakfast and lunch, the easiest way to achieve this is implement the practice of only having two meals a day and eliminate snacks between meals and dinner. If we set a schedule example, it would be something like this: if you eat breakfast at seven o'clock in the morning and eat at two o'clock in the afternoon, you do not eat anything else from then until seven o'clock in the morning next day, except water, coffee, or tea. You thus maintain a 16-hour fasting period.

Alternatively, eating Breakfast at 7.00 am and then a light dinner at seven in the afternoon and not eating anything else until breakfast at seven in the morning can be limited to a 12-hour fast window initially and then work on building up to a 16-hour fasting period, if going straight into a 16 hour fast is too complicated, to start with.

Other methods include occasional fasting periods longer than two or three days or intermittent alternate fasting days. The fasting day greatly reduces the number of calories (one or two meals to a total of 500 calories), and the next day you eat when your stomach tells you too.'

Ketogenic Diet

I wanted to mention this type of diet which is a high fat and low carbohydrate feeding system and works similarly to intermittent fasting. This diet causes the body to adjust its metabolism to burn fat for energy instead of sugar. Anyway, it needs to be clear that it is not about eating just any kind of fat; you still need to prioritize healthy fats like coconut or olive oil, avocados, cow butter, or nuts.

Moreover, the carbohydrates that are ingested must come from vegetables to add vitamins and fiber. The ketone bodies produced when fat is used as fuel induce autophagy, with its nervous system protective functions. This particular diet has been shown to be extremely effective when combined with Intermittent Fasting.

Exercise as A Trigger for Autophagy

Practicing exercise is a way to create "healthy" pressure for the body because tissues that need to be healed to become more resilient are damaged. This will trigger the process we are considering.

What type of exercise is recommended for this purpose is not yet clear, although intensive exercise is probably the most suitable. Through 30 minutes of exercise, this cycle is necessary to unleash the process in the tissues of the musculoskeletal system.

Before you start eating, you can combine exercise with fasting and perform your exercise routine, although it is not clear whether it works better after your first meal or after, this does depend on each individual's situation.

The Difference between Cleaning Diets and Fasting

The body as a recycling plant

When we eat, the body uses the nutrient energy to function normally and in order to reconstruct. The cells of your skin, hair, lungs, liver, and the rest of your body are regenerated daily as a result of the proteins we take with the food.

On the contrary, when nutrients are missing, our body goes into catabolism: it is dedicated to breaking them down instead of building tissues. Muscles are the tissues first dismantled to use those proteins whenever possible. But the body is not stupid when it comes to recycling, and it chooses the cells that have already been aged or damaged. You use parts of the scrap.

This process is called autophagy and is as simple as yeasts already present in living organisms.

mTOR is an acronym for rapamycin target in mammals and it is the molecule that regulates the balance between cell reconstruction or recycling, it is in fact a relatively new discovery that was released in 1993.

The system is quite complex, but if mTOR is inhibited, it increases autophagy and apoptosis (cellular suicide). On the contrary, if mTOR increases uncontrollably, we have some sort of cell-building immovable bubble or, in other words, cancer. It has been shown that mTOR is involved in breast, prostate, kidney, melanoma, bladder, and brain tumors. It is also suspected that when mTOR does not work well, the accumulation of defective cells causes aging and neurodegenerative diseases.

How then to stimulate recycling in the body? A good way is to stop eating once in a while.

The short-term fast (between 24 and 72 hours) produces mTOR inhibition and activates autophagy, the true cleansing. Fasting has shown incredibly positive effects in the laboratory:

1. Slow down aging

2. Reduce inflammation, which increases with stress and excess sugar in the diet

3. Increase autophagy in the brain, which prevents Alzheimer's

4. Prevent and treat diabetes

5. Reduce obesity, hypertension, asthma, and rheumatoid arthritis

Some of these experiments have obtained similar results by reducing calories without reaching full fast. But in other aspects, eating less is not the same as stop eating altogether. For starters, it will cost you much more.

Eat little or not eat anything

Some years ago, one Doctor, in particular, made us think that fats were bad for forty years (by selecting the data he felt like from a variety of studies). This particular doctor was also the author of a controversial experiment in which the volunteers were on a regime where they lost a quarter of their weight and which had a number of serious side effects for the subjects, such as suffering from depression, loss of sexual desire, antisocial behavior, and cognitive abilities loss. Their basal metabolisms dropped, and, worse, during the experiment, they were hungry all the time and became totally obsessed with food.

It is extremely difficult not to eat anything. Conversely, it has been proven that hunger on the second day disappears when the fast is total. This is due to ghrelin, the hormone that arouses appetite, and which is the opposite of leptin, which tells us, unfortunately, not early enough that we've eaten enough. Ghrelin decreases during fasting and with it the sensation of hunger.

Fasting does not produce a decrease in basal metabolism and if that was not enough; it also increases it during the first four days. That is, the body absorbs more energy at rest. It also affects the ability of the body to control blood sugar and insulin levels. In an experiment with obese women, it was found that when comparing intermittent fasting two days a week with a calorie-restrictive diet, in both cases, the levels of cholesterol, triglycerides, and blood pressure were reduced. However, insulin sensitivity increased much more with fasting.

Fasting seems to specifically affect insulin levels. It will go up every time we eat carbohydrates or insulin protein. However, in full fasting (drinking water only), insulin levels drop after about 24 hours, and the body starts using fat as fuel. That's not at all new. A century ago, fasting was used for the treatment of diabetes before the discovery of insulin.

Using maple syrup, honey, or fruit juice increases insulin levels again in detox diets and stops our body from burning fat for several hours. Moreover, so-called reactive hypoglycemia can be caused by insulin spikes. Within a few hours of eating, blood sugar levels drop suddenly, and the feeling of hunger appears, along with nervousness, irritability, and difficulty concentrating.

Even using these types of diets to lose weight isn't a good idea. One of these purges' results was observed with lemon water and honey for four days in one study. The effects saw a drop in body weight and triglycerides. However, something odd occurred;

although the weight of the participants decreased, the percentage of body fat remained the same because the loss of fat was followed by a reduction of muscle mass. It is always a bad idea to lose muscle.

A full speed fast for a day or two can have beneficial effects, but there are risks and involved without medical supervision, and prolonged fasting for more than 72 hours should never occur. The risk increases even more significantly, when illnesses like gout, stomach reflux, chronic kidney disease, type 1 diabetes, or eating disorders are present or occur.

We also need to bear in mind that 30% of the water is obtained from food, so it is even more important to drink more water than normal during fasting to avoid dehydration complications. Another point to remember, is that It can be uncomfortable at best and dangerous at worst to eat a lot at once after a fast. It is better to begin drinking juices or eating fruit and to start to introduce other foods gradually.

Finally, remember that many of the significant fasting benefits can be obtained by intermittent fasting, which only lasts 24 hours.

What Is All This Based On?

To help us to better understand all of this we need to look at mTOR and how it affects the Human Body. The human body has a special protein called mammalian target of rapamycin (**mTOR** for short). Many experts now refer to this as the muscle-building gene.

mTOR signaling in tumorigenesis

mTOR signaling pathway deregulation is one of the most commonly observed pathological changes in human cancers. To this end, oncogenic activation of the mTOR signaling pathway contributes to cancer cell growth, proliferation, and survival, highlighting the potential of targeting mTOR oncogenic pathway members as an effective cancer strategy.

Autophagy and aging; the importance of maintaining "clean" cells

It has been proven that dietary caloric restriction and antilipolytic agents efficiently stimulate autophagy in older rodents.

The mammalian target of rapamycin at the crossroad between cognitive aging and Alzheimer's disease

Suppressing the target of rapamycin in mammals (mTOR) in several species increases lifespan and life expectancy. Several studies have linked changes in mTOR signaling to age-dependent cognitive impairment and Alzheimer's disease pathogenesis.

Calorie restriction: decelerating mTOR-driven aging from cells to organisms (including humans).

Various studies suggest that aging is partly due to the detection of nutrients by the TOR network (target of rapamycin). CR disables the TOR route, delaying aging and delaying aging diseases. Human beings are no exception, and CR should increase people's maximum and healthy lifespan to the same extent as other mammals.

Alternate-day fasting protects the rat heart against age-induced inflammation and fibrosis by inhibiting oxidative damage and NF-kB activation.

These data support the hypothesis that this type of dietary restriction protects against age-related fibrosis, at least partially, by reducing inflammation and oxidative damage. This protection may be considered a factor in age-related disease prevention with the evolution of sclerotic.

Short-term fasting induces profound neuronal autophagy

A wide variety of data lead us to believe that intermittent fasting could be a quick, healthy, and economical way of promoting this possible neuronal therapeutic response; this was born out in a 2-group study on the effects of intermittent or constant energy restriction on weight loss and risk factors of metabolic disease: with a randomized study of young women who were overweight.

Reductions in insulin fasting and insulin resistance were modest in both groups but were greater with intermittent Fasting energy restrictions than with the constant restrictions on energy.

Fasting: molecular mechanisms and clinical applications

In rodents, periodic or intermittent fasting protects against diabetes, cancers, heart disease, and neurodegeneration, while in humans, it helps reduce obesity, hypertension, asthma, and rheumatoid arthritis.

Resting energy expenditure in short-term starvation is increased as a direct result of an increase in serum norepinephrine.

The resting energy expenditure increases in early starvation, accompanied by an increase in plasma norepinephrine. This increase in norepinephrine appears to be due to decreased serum glucose and maybe the initial signal of fasting metabolic changes.

The Treatment of Diabetes Mellitus

That period of under nutrition to help treat diabetes will probably be recognized within a few months of the commencement of a fasting program.

Hypoglycemia is reactive.

Patients with this condition's relationship to meals can often be characterized by the ingestion of excessive amounts of refined carbohydrates.

Does a short-term lemon honey juice fast affect lipid profile and body composition in healthy individuals?

One study showed a significant weight reduction, body mass index (BMI), fat mass (FM), free fat mass (FMM), and total serum triglycerides (TSTG) but with an insignificant reduction in fat percentage and total serum cholesterol compared to the starting baseline.

CHAPTER TEN

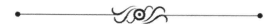

COMBINING INTERMITTENT FASTING WITH CYCLIC NUTRITIONAL KETOSIS

During what is called the "feedback" phase, most of these rejuvenating and regenerating benefits occur, not in the "starvation" phase. The same applies to nutritional ketosis, which, when performed in lapses, produces the greatest benefits.

Some of the metabolic health parameters that have not improved significantly have been visceral fat mass, diastolic blood pressure, LDL cholesterol, HDL cholesterol, fasting glucose, triglycerides, and fasting insulin. Cyclic ketosis provides many of the same health benefits associated with intermittent fasting, and when the two are combined, most people experience significant improvements in their health and weight loss.

For thousands of years, fasting has been implemented to keep us healthy, and it is the most effective metabolic intervention I know. It not only upregulates autophagy and mitophagy — which are the natural processes of cleaning required to maximize cell regeneration and function — but it also activates stem cell development. Similarly, cyclical withdrawal from food accompanied by feedback (recovery) promotes major biosynthesis of the mitochondria.

Even evidence suggests that fasting may help prevent or even reverse dementia, eliminating toxic waste from the body. Lowering insulin levels also increases other important hormones, including growth hormone (known as "the fitness hormone"), which is important for muscle development and overall vitality.

Most of these rejuvenating and regenerating benefits occur during the feedback phase, not the "starvation" phase. The same goes for nutritional ketosis, which produces the greatest benefits when done in lapses.

Fasting Is A Powerful Tool for Rejuvenation and Overall Health

Research shows that fasting is a powerful lifestyle tool to combat obesity, insulin resistance, and related health problems, including cancer. The reason is that your body starts breaking down and recycling old proteins, including beta-amyloid protein, in the brain, which is believed to contribute to Alzheimer's disease when the autophagy process decreases.

Later, growth hormone levels increase during the feedback phase, which leads to the reconstruction of new proteins and cells. In other words, it reactivates and accelerates the body's natural renewal cycle. Although fasting with just water can be extremely beneficial for people with type 2 diabetes and/or overweight, the implementation may be difficult.

Fortunately, research has confirmed that similar (although not as profound) results can be obtained by intermittent fasting; that is, by following a feeding schedule that allows you to fast for at least 16 hours a day and consume all your meals within eight consecutive hours. Alternatively, there are other intermittent fasting programs in which you reduce your calories dramatically for a certain number of days while eating normally for the rest of the week.

To Optimize Your Health, Combine Intermittent Fasting with Cyclic Nutritional Ketosis

Therefore, while this study presents intermittent fasting as a successful weight-loss method, it emphasizes the importance of combining intermittent fasting with cyclic nutritional ketosis for optimum effect

The ketogenic diet provides many of the same health benefits related to intermittent fasting and fasting (mentioned above). When implemented together, most people may experience significant improvements in their health -including weight loss, which is more than just an inevitable side effect of the metabolic improvements. For example, the benefits of eating a ketogenic diet include.

Further insulin resistance, it is important to avoid resistance to insulin, type 2 diabetes, and related diseases. Studies have shown that sufferers of diabetes on a ketogenic diet can significantly reduce their dependency on diabetes drugs. Many even reversed their diabetes successfully. In addition, because dementia and insulin resistance are closely related, having a healthy insulin level can also reduce the risk of Alzheimer's disease.

Increased muscle mass Ketones are structurally similar to branched-chain amino acids. As they tend to preferentially metabolize, they reserve any branched-chain amino acid and stimulate mass muscle development.

Less inflammation - The body is designed to use sugar and fat as fuel sources with metabolic versatility. Nonetheless, it is better to use fats because they contain fewer reactive oxygen species and secondary free radicals when they are burned. Instead, removing sugar from food greatly reduces your risk of chronic inflammation.

Low cancer risk. It is now thought by a number of researchers that while cyclic ketosis is considered to be a novel treatment, it could dramatically reduce the risk of becoming another cancer statistic simply because cancer cells would lack the metabolic ability to use ketones to fulfill their energy needs compared to normal cells.

Once the body performs nutritional ketosis, cancer cells no longer have an available food source and die of starvation before generating problems. Longevity Ketosis prevents protein breakdown, which is one reason you can survive a long time without feeding.

Like caloric restriction (fasting), ketones also help sanitize immune cell's malfunction and decrease IGF-1, which regulates growth pathways and growth genes and plays an important role in aging autophagy and mitophagy.

Also, ketone metabolism increases the negative reduction-oxidation (redox) potential of the NAD redox coenzyme family of molecules, which helps control oxidative damage by increasing NADPH levels and promoting the transcription of enzymes from antioxidant pathways through activating FOXO3a. In saying that, ketone metabolism effectively decreases oxidative damage, which translates into better health and longevity.

Also, the lack of sugar helps explain why the ketogenic diet is related to longevity. Sugar is a powerful accelerator of aging and premature death, partly because it activates two genes known as Ras and PKA, accelerating the aging process.

A third reason is related to the fact that the mTOR pathway, which has been shown to play an important role in longevity, is inhibited by both caloric and intermittent fasting.

If you are trying to lose weight, eating a ketogenic diet is one of the best ways to do this, as it helps to eliminate body fat. For one study, a low-carb ketogenic diet and a low-fat diet were followed by 16 overweight test subjects. The researchers observed after 24 weeks that the low-carb group lost more weight (9.4 kg; 20.7 pounds) than the low-fat group (4.8 kg; 10.5 pounds).

How to Implement Cyclic Ketosis and Fasting?

Fasting and metabolic ketosis both have many of the same advantages, and when applied in lapses, both work at their best. Many experts in both fields agree that cyclic ketosis and intermittent fasting are an almost unbeatable combination that can fully optimize health benefits by implementing them together.

Although the "Fat for Fuel" work principle provides more detailed information, this book contains a summary of how these two strategies can be implemented as a combined health program: implement an intermittent schedule of fasting. In an extremely basic approach, by eating all your food regardless of whether it's breakfast and lunch or lunch and dinner-every day within 8 hours, and fast for the remaining 16 hours.

If all this is new to you and you think the idea of making changes in your diet and eating habits is very daunting, just continue with a regular diet for a short time when beginning to practice Intermittent Fasting and then once you have successfully done that you can continue to implement the ketogenic diet followed by the cyclic portion (step 3). You may feel more comfortable knowing that you can cycle daily with some of your favorite healthy carbohydrates once you hit phase 3.

Consider increasing the rate by fasting for a couple of days of water alone regularly if you want to maximize the benefits even more significantly by fasting alone. Personally, I do these three to four times a year to kick start the process and then Gradually increase to a gentle Intermittent Fasting point (12 hours) before increasing to a point where you can fast for longer periods a day (16 hours) and consume your two meals in a smaller number of hours to facilitate the process further. It won't be too hard to perform a one day or two-day water fast after having been used to a smaller feeding window.

Change to a ketogenic diet until measurable ketone levels can be produced. The trick is in three parts: first, limit net carbohydrates (total carbohydrates without fiber) from 20 to 50 grams a day; second, replace lost carbohydrates with healthy fats, so you can get between 50 and 85 percent of your daily calories via fat.

And third, restrict your protein consumption to half a gram of protein per pound of lean body mass. There are a number of tools on the internet to assist you to do this, I personally find it helpful to see a visual representation of how much this actually is as it can be quite hard to work out.

Several examples of healthy fat sources are avocados, coconut oil, fatty fish animal omega-3 fats, butter, unprocessed nuts (macadamia nuts and pecans are suitable as they are high in nutritious and low protein fat), seeds, olives and olive oil, pasture-fed animal products, MCT oil, unprocessed cocoa butter and organic egg yolks from country chickens.

Both trans fats and polyunsaturated vegetable oils are highly processed and could cause you more harm than a carbohydrate overload, so just because a food is "high in fat" doesn't mean you should eat it.

Keep a strict eye proportions of net carbohydrates, fats, and proteins until ketosis is reached and fat is burned for fuel by your body. You can easily purchase the ketosis test strips that can be used to verify that you have started the process, which is described as a range of ketones in the blood from 0.5 to 3.0 mol / L.

Note that when it comes to these nutrient proportions, reliability is an important issue. Too many net carbohydrates prevent ketosis from being effectively performed as the body uses any available glucose the first instance because it is a much faster fuel to utilize.

Since the amount of fat, net carbohydrates, and protein in each food is virtually impossible to estimate reliably, you should make sure that you have some simple measuring and monitoring devices, such as Kitchen scales, measuring spoons, cups etc.

Once you've confirmed you're in the process of ketosis, it is good practice to pause and restart the cycles of ketosis. This can easily be achieved by including higher net carbohydrate numbers once or twice a week. As a general recommendation, on high carbohydrate days, triple the number of net carbohydrates. Consider the possibility that it might take you from a couple of weeks to months before your body can effectively burn fat again.

Again, by pausing and restarting nutritional ketosis, you will maximize the biological benefits of cell renewal and regeneration while minimizing the potential inconvenience and side effects of continuous ketosis.

CHAPTER ELEVEN

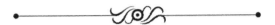

LOSE FAT WITHOUT LOSING MUSCLE

The reduction in calories increases the metabolic rate and energy use, so the body must use the additional energy in your body to compensate. You can say this, but it will ideally be your ugly stored fat. On the other hand, it is still muscle tissue, although it is lower in weight.

Fat is good, too. The research shows that body fat loss without adequate muscle building results in loss of lean body mass. Muscle gain and excess fat do not go hand in hand, meaning that it might result in a less desirable shape regardless of what you lose. As far as we know, a body will have to tap into accumulated resources to carry out the everyday activities you have to do to stay alive. More generally, it may mean fat and muscle, depending on the definition.

If you choose to accept it, your mission is to do everything possible to improve the fat loss proportion: protect the muscle as much as possible and basically instruct your body to maintain ALL your muscles and ONLY burn body fat, (this is especially important for women over the age of 40). But the question is, HOW? I thought you'd never ask.

Here Are What Experts Consider to be The Eight Best Ways to Lose Fat WITHOUT Losing Muscle

1. Eat enough protein

The most important dietary necessity for preserving muscle is an adequate daily intake of protein. It's not the meal schedule, the nutrients, the exact size of your caloric deficit, the quality of the food you consume (more about that later), or anything else relevant to the diet.

Nutritionally speaking, it is about eating enough protein every day to lose fat without losing muscle. Even in the absence of a proper weight training routine, a larger amount of weight you lose will be body fat instead of muscle mass due to increased protein intake. Therefore, any diet's first step to preserve muscles is to obtain the ideal amount of protein for the day. The question is, what is ideal?

Well, research and real-world experience have shown that something in the range of 0.8-1.3g of protein per pound of your current body weight is the optimal point for people with this goal. Full details here: How much protein do I need per day?

2. Maintain strength levels

And now, for anyone who wants to lose weight without losing muscle, we have the most important training requirement. Simply put, maintaining your current strength levels is the primary training stimulus needed to maintain the muscle.

Do you know how to reinforce yourself (also known as the progressive overload principle) slowly? This is what tells your body to start the process of muscle building. Okay, maintaining your current strength levels (also known as power, also known as barbell weight) on a diet to lose fat is what now tells your body to hold your muscles.

That's why the stupid myth of lifting heavier weights to build muscle but then lifting lighter weights (for higher repetitions) if you want to lose fat, lose weight, and tone up is the WORST thing you can believe in trying to avoid muscle loss. If you want to preserve the muscle, you lift heavy weight to build muscle and raise the same heavyweight.

If you start lifting lighter weights intentionally while having a caloric deficit, your body thinks essentially: "Hmmm, it seems we just need to lift lighter weights now. I guess you don't need all that muscle that I developed to be able to lift heavyweights. It's time to start burning it for energy instead of body fat!

3. Reduce the volume and/or frequency of weight training

A caloric deficit is an energy deficit. While losing any body fat amount is fantastic (and necessary), it is a bit bad for everything related to training (recovery, ability to work, volume tolerance, performance, etc.).

What this means is that the training routine you were (or would be) using with great success to build muscle, increase strength, or make any other positive improvements in your body under normal circumstances (where there is no deficit) has the potential to be too much for your body to handle and recover optimally in the current state of energy deficiency. Do you know what this scenario usually leads to, one in which you are not recovering enough? A loss of strength. And do you know what a loss of strength will lead to, especially in a caloric deficit? A muscle loss.

The key training requirement to maintain muscle is simply to maintain strength. If you are using a training routine from which you are not recovering properly, the opposite will happen. This is something I have learned through the years, along with many others. The louder volume, the 4–6-day training routine that appeared to be fine when those extra beneficial calories were present now is the reason why things get harder, you're weakening, the repetitions are decreasing, the weight of the bar needs to be reduced, and your phase of fat loss (also known as the cutting phase) ends with the muscle loss and strength you should have lost.

How can you avoid all this easily? Fortunately, it's easy through changing the weight training regimen to counteract the fall in recovery resulting in a caloric deficit. That could mean reducing your existing training volume, or by reducing training frequency (for example, using a 3-day training routine instead of a 5-day training routine), or a combination of both.

If you need help with this, there are a number of articles available that establish how to make these adjustments so that you can easily turn any smart workout routine to build muscle into one that is ideal for maintaining it or check with your professional trainer or medical professional.

A possible exception to this would be beginners. They should already be using a routine for low-volume all-around beginners designed intelligently.

4. Get proper nutrition before and after training

As mentioned, recovery, work capacity, volume tolerance, and overall training performance, in general, these deteriorate as a result of a prolonged caloric deficit, even if you haven't heard about it, the

69

whole concept of pre- and post-training nutrition is based on improving these aspects of training and recovery.

That makes the meals you eat before and after your workouts just as important (possibly even more) when your goal is to lose fat without losing muscle instead of simply building that muscle in the first place. So, what should you eat during these meals? Simple: consume a good amount of protein and carbohydrates within 1-2 hours before and after your workout. There is no need to make it more complicated than that.

5. Don't reduce calories too much

As we expect everyone to understand now, to lose any body fat, you must create a caloric deficit. That means you will need to reduce your calorie intake below the maintenance level so that stored body fat can be burned for energy.

The point is that this deficit can be classified as small, moderate, or large, depending on how low the maintenance goes and how much it reduces your daily calorie intake. While each degree of the deficit has its pros and cons, a moderate deficit of approximately 20% below the maintenance level tends to be ideal for most people.

Why not a major deficit? Why not reduce calories much more and make fat loss even faster? Well, apart from that, it worsens metabolic deceleration, hormonal problems, hunger, mood, sleep, libido, lethargy (and more), It is simply more difficult to maintain. Another major disadvantage of a great Caloric deficit is that it will have the greatest negative impact on training and recovery. And that means that reducing calories too much will increase the potential for strength loss and muscle loss and for that reason alone, it is recommended that most people stay with a moderate deficit. Those who are already quite slim and looking to be thinner can do much better with an even smaller deficit.

6. Avoid excessive amounts of cardio (or just do nothing)

All this goes back to what I already mentioned several times about reducing recovery due to calorie reduction. For this reason, ALL the exercise you are doing (not only weight training but also cardio) may need to be reduced or adjusted to some extent to compensate for this and help prevent muscle loss.

Tips and Care to Burn Fat with Intermittent Fasting

If you intend to follow one of the intermittent fasting methods to lose fat while gaining muscle mass in hypertrophy training, here are some tips to help you succeed in this task.

1. Frequent training

The frequency of bodybuilding training is important as it can help you maintain muscles during intermittent fasting. Several studies show that weight training is responsible for preventing muscle loss when following a weight loss diet.

A specific study on intermittent fasting examined the combination of intermittent fasting and weight training three days a week for eight weeks. The scientists divided 34 very experienced men in weight training into two groups: one of them had intermittent fasting of 8 hours of feeding followed by 16 hours of fasting, while the other group followed a normal diet.

Both groups consumed the same number of calories and the same amount of protein per day, changing only the frequency and time of meals. At the end of the study, the researchers realized that none of the groups showed a loss of lean mass or strength. However,

71

the group that followed the intermittent fast lost 1.6 kg of fat, while the other group showed no changes in the macronutrients' body composition. This shows that frequent hypertrophy training during intermittent fasting can help maintain muscles and cause good fat loss as long as protein needs are met.

Also, other research indicates that fasting on alternate days with approximately 25 to 40 minutes of aerobic exercises, such as cycling or elliptical training, for example, three times a week, can also help maintain muscle mass during weight loss. Therefore, the general practice of exercise is essential to maintain the muscles during intermittent fasting.

2. Limited protein synthesis

Since the feeding window is restricted, it can be more difficult to overcome your protein target. In order to increase protein synthesis for muscle mass, it is recommended to eat approximately 3 to 4 servings of protein per day with an interval of approximately 3 hours between servings. In intermittent fasting, this is not possible, which makes lean mass synthesis a bit more challenging.

3. The best time to train

There is a discussion about the best time to perform physical activities during intermittent fasting. A 4-week study of 20 participants looked at women who were not fasting and another group that was fasting. Study participants exercised three days a week for an hour on a treadmill at a comfortable pace. It was observed that both groups had the same weight and fat loss, and neither of them underwent changes in the percentage of lean mass.

According to this study, it does not seem to make a difference if the exercise is performed on an empty stomach or not. What often happens is that physical performance can be reduced by doing intense fasting exercises. Therefore, if you need to have excellent performance, especially in bodybuilding exercises, it is indicated that you do the exercises after eating and avoid very intense fasting activities. If you choose to train your fasting muscles, get a protein source right after your session to ensure good muscle recovery.

4. Weight loss control

Experts say that the faster the weight loss, the greater the chances of losing lean mass. Therefore, it is not indicated that you follow a very drastic diet to lose weight if your goal is to maintain muscles. Do not reduce your caloric intake so much at once with intermittent fasting and maintain your weight loss rate of 400 to 900 grams per week to ensure no muscle loss.

5. Proper nutrition

Nutrition is particularly important regardless of the diet followed. The composition of the diet is especially important to keep the muscles fasting. Therefore, it is important to eat quality protein to preserve lean mass during fat burning promoted by intermittent fasting. Consumption of at least 0.7 grams of protein per kg of body weight is indicated daily. It is also important to choose nutritious foods containing dietary fiber, healthy fats essential for brain health, and good carbohydrates.

6. Supplements

You can also opt for dietary supplements to help maintain muscles during intermittent fasting. Supplements should be taken during the feeding window to avoid impairing fasting. The most important include sources of protein, BCAA, and creatine. Although supplementation is unnecessary if you get the protein you need through diet, supplementation may be interesting to ensure protein and other nutrients during the short daily feeding window. Also, protein supplements can improve physical performance and facilitate mass gain.

Intermittent fasting is an excellent diet to promote weight loss, especially fat burning. Athletes who always seek to reduce fat and increase lean mass can benefit greatly from intermittent fasting to alter body composition. Although there are many myths about muscle loss during fasting, no muscle loss is observed when combined with good nutrition and regular physical activity.

Suppose you have difficulty gaining lean mass and struggling to achieve your daily protein and other macronutrients' daily goal. In that case, intermittent fasting may not be the best option to gain mass.

CHAPTER TWELVE

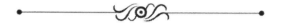

SUPERFOODS FOR WOMEN OVER 40

As we age, we need to take more and more seriously the foods we eat and our nutritional requirements to maintain a healthy metabolism and fat levels. Choosing the right foods for women over 40 will give our body vitamins and nutrients to ensure that we maintain good health for a longer time. Here are some of the superfoods that are especially important for women over 40.

Raspberries and blueberries

In general, all berries are suitable foods for women. However, for women in our 40's, these two types have specific benefits. Raspberries contain special phytochemicals that fight some cancer cells but are also high in fiber.

Blueberries, on the other hand, are a powerful antioxidant that helps the body to fight various inflammations, bacteria, and viruses. You can use them in all kinds of cheesecakes, milk with honey, homemade ice cream, or decorating salads or desserts.

Eggs

Make a fluffy omelet or boil eggs. No matter how you prepare them, they are still healthy. Yolks contain fat that will keep you full for longer, and the choline content helps burn belly fat. Eggs are a real super-food for women over 40.

Avocado

This fruit has an extremely high content of healthy fats, which can help reduce bad cholesterol levels. On top of that, they are also extremely filling and will keep you full for a longer time.

Chickpeas

Chickpeas are remarkably high in fiber, and according to some studies, they also support hormone levels during the period leading up to and including menopause. In addition to eating them alone, you can mix them with different sauces or prepare a delicious hummus by mixing them with tahini, lemon juice, and salt. You can also make delicious falafels or other vegetarian meatballs.

Carrots

Do you want your skin to be smooth? Then you need to get vitamin A. And what more natural way to do this than eating carrots. Also, it will help keep your vision sharp for longer. Do not give up carrot salad. And if you like to eat sweets, choose a carrot cake.

Apples

Frequent consumption of this sweet fruit reduces the risk of developing various diseases of the cardiovascular system. Make apple pancakes or plain baked apples with honey. And you can also put the apples in a tasty and nutritious salad.

Honey

Honey contains high levels of a variety of nutrients. Forget about artificial sweeteners and add a little honey to your coffee or tea. It contains minerals such as copper, iron, magnesium, manganese, phosphorus, potassium, sodium, and zinc. They strengthen your immune system and improve the overall condition of the body. It is among the best foods for women over 40.

Olive oil

Olive oil supports the body's activity in several areas. One of the most important of these, is that it supports the unlocking and operation of fat-soluble vitamins A, E, D, and K, which are found in many types of lettuce and other salad vegetables. Olive oil is also associated with weight loss and the prevention of heart disease

Anti-Aging Foods for Women Over 40

1 - Pomegranate seeds

It is one of the healthiest fruits. Its antioxidant activity appears to be even greater than that of green tea. Also, they are rich in vitamin C, which protects our body from free radical damage and reduces inflammation levels. These fruits contain a compound called punicalagin, an antioxidant that can help preserve the skin's collagen, slowing the signs of aging and acting as an anti-aging food. They also help to protect the skin from damage from the sun. What is more, many researchers suggest that different parts of the pomegranate can work together to repair damaged skin and increase collagen production.

2 - Avocado

These are rich in fatty acids, which fight inflammation and promote soft and flexible skin. They also contain various essential nutrients that can prevent aging, including vitamins K, C, E, and A, B complex, and potassium. The high vitamin A content in avocados can eliminate dead cells, leaving beautiful and glowing skin. Its carotenoid content can also help block toxins and damage from the sun's rays and help protect against skin cancer. Besides, avocados contain unique compounds called polyhydroxylated fatty alcohols. They can fight inflammation, protect your skin from the sun, and help repair damaged DNA. Their high content of monounsaturated fat, and the antioxidants lutein and zeaxanthin, provide additional protection to the skin and DNA.

3 - Watercress

Watercress is an anti-aging food that acts as an internal antiseptic, increasing the circulation and distribution of minerals to

78

all cells, resulting in greater oxygenation of the skin. Rich in antioxidants, watercress neutralizes harmful free radicals, reducing fine lines and fine wrinkles. Watercress isothiocyanates can also prevent skin cancer. These compounds interfere with malignant cells and restore normal cell function.

4 - Red Pepper

Red peppers are rich in antioxidants called carotenoids and vitamin C, which helps in collagen production. Carotenoids are plant pigments responsible for the colors red, yellow, and orange and are present in many fruits and vegetables. They have various anti-inflammatory properties and can help protect your skin from sunlight, pollution, and environmental toxins.

5 - Blueberry

Blueberries are rich in vitamins A, C, and anthocyanin. These antioxidants fight free radicals and protect our skin from exposure to the sun, stress, and pollution, moderating the inflammatory response and preventing the loss of collagen, which can cause damage to the skin over time and accelerate the aging process. Blueberries also contain significant amounts of zinc and iron, both of which are skin-friendly elements.

6 - Papaya

Papaya is an anti-aging food rich in vitamins A, C, K, E, and B complex, calcium, potassium, magnesium, and phosphorus. It is well known as a source of antioxidants that helps fight free radicals, delay's the signs of aging, reduces wrinkles and expression lines and can decrease acne (especially in adolescents) and melasma.

7 - Spinach

It is a super moisturizer full of antioxidants, which help to oxygenate and replenish the whole body. It is also rich in vitamins A, C, E, K, magnesium, heme iron and lutein. The high vitamin C content of this green leaf increases collagen production to keep the skin firm. Vitamin A promotes strong, shiny hair, while vitamin K helps to reduce inflammation in cells.

8 - Almond

These are a great vitamin E source, which helps repair skin tissue, retain moisture and protects from UV rays. Almonds contain omega-3 fatty acids, an anti-inflammatory that helps strengthen the skin's cell membranes against damage from the sun's rays and give the skin a shine while preserving its natural barrier. In addition, they also provide fiber, essential fats, and proteins. They are responsible for making the skin soft and flexible and giving it a natural shine and a smoother appearance. So, if you haven't added almonds to your diet yet, do it now to promote naturally glowing and healthy skin.

9 - Seasonings and Spices

Spices do more than just add flavor to food. They contain several compounds that can have beneficial health effects. Research suggests that some spices can even help your skin to look younger. This is the case, especially with cinnamon, which has been shown to increase collagen production and has increased skin firmness and elasticity. Besides, ginger contains gingerol and this compound has anti-inflammatory effects that can help prevent age spots, which develop due to exposure to the sun.

10 - Sweet Potato

The orange color of sweet potatoes comes from an antioxidant called beta carotene, which is converted into vitamin A. It helps restore the skin's elasticity, it promotes the renewal of dead cells, and it contributes to smooth and healthy-looking skin. Sweet potatoes are also rich in vitamin C and vitamin E, both of which are crucially important for keeping your skin healthy, glowing, and supple. Vitamin C especially helps to increase collagen, which strengthens the skin. The antioxidants in sweet potatoes are also responsible for the skin's natural glow. This tuber is also a rich source of anthocyanin that helps prevent dark spots, keeping free radical activity under control.

11 - Broccoli

Broccoli is another of these Amazing of the anti-aging, Super foods. Skin appearance does not only improve but this vegetable also boosts your immunity. Since broccoli is a source of antioxidants and nutrients like vitamin C and minerals like copper and zinc, broccoli helps to maintain healthy skin. This also means that it also protects the skin against infections, as well as maintaining the skin's natural glow. Besides, Vitamin C which helps in the production of collagen, making the skin look younger. Broccoli also contains a substance called glucoraphanin which convert's to sulforaphane, which helps repair the skin, making it healthier. Thus, eating broccoli renews your skin more quickly and gives your complexion a beautiful natural glow.

Tips to Slow Aging

The idea is not to deprive ourselves of everything we like but to improve our quality of life by thinking about our present and future nutritional needs intelligently. The human being can adapt to any change; by incorporating healthy habits and we can make easy changes to improve our lifestyle.

Any good change is for the better.

What we need to remember is that diseases and damage occur when cells (e.g., cardiovascular, cerebral, ocular) are inflamed and deteriorate due to lack of food, poor nutrition, insufficient oxygenation, and excess toxins, resulting in cell pressure and accelerated aging.

Here I give you some easy to adopt, simple and economic recommendations, which can bring us great benefits.

1. Continuous hydration. Water is the main nutrient essential for living. In our bodies, it is about 50 to 60 percent. Foods (such as fruits and vegetables) provide 20% of the water we need; an adult or older adult should drink between 1.5 and 2 liters per day.

Infusions (e.g., chamomile, lemon verbena, anise), natural soda (e.g., pineapple, apple, lemonade), or pure water are considered moisturizing liquids. It is important to avoid soda's, box juices, or artificial liquids.

Water makes it possible for all cells in our body to perform their functions better; it improves blood pressure and heart effort, protects the kidneys, reduces pain in general, improves visual acuity and mental capacity. Older adults are often thirsty; however, water requirements are not always maintained. Remember that it is important to drink water, so you do not thirst and to maintain optimum body condition.

2. Fresh and natural food. Food is the energy that enters our body; the better the quality, the more vitality we will have. Peas, fruits, and vegetables in general, fish, nuts (such as chocolate, pecans, almonds), tubers (such as rice, cassava, sweet potatoes), cereals (such as oats, quinoa), essential oils (such as olive oil, Sacha inch) is preferable. The key is a varied diet, well-balanced, and full of variety and colors.

As their additives return acid to the cells, we must avoid processed foods, canned, or foods containing preservatives or dyes as these predispose to stress and cell aging. We increase our immunity or defense capacity with a well-balanced diet, which prevents chronic degenerative diseases or exacerbates existing diseases.

3. Physical activity. The longer we remain active functionally, the better. We can do the workouts we like most, as we get older less high impact exercises like swimming, singing, yoga, cycling, walking, Pilates and Tai Chi, tend to suit us better. It is always good to combine different types of exercises and preferably outdoors and to vary the times. Ideally, spread them over the week for 150 minutes in total Increasing physical activity in time and with varying levels of intensity and remember intensity depends on each individual's tolerance, make sure you seek advice from your Healthcare provider before starting on an exercise program.

Physical activity is crucially important at all ages, as it improves oxygenation, cardiovascular function, muscle mass, prevents falling, metabolic problems, and it plays an important part of the treatment of depression.

4. Good night's rest. It is recommended to sleep between 6 to 8 hours; however, the idea is to get up with the feeling of having had a restful sleep. The dream state resets the memory and recharges the energies for our daily activities.

5. Breathing and oxygenation. We breathe about 16 times a minute, but very seldom do we focus on doing it properly. To properly ventilate our lungs, it is important to expand our thoracic cavity and lower the diaphragm (main respiratory muscle). Oxygen prevents free radicals or toxic substances from accumulating as they stress our cells and age them.

Note that cancers develop in sugar-rich environments, in salt, with little oxygen, and without water. Therefore, it is necessary to keep well-oxygenated, hydrated, and to eat adequate nutritious food to prevent oncological diseases.

6. Emotional intelligence. Is the ability to become aware of our emotions and those of others and it helps us to respond appropriately to them to achieve positive effects. It allows us to resolve conflicts in a better way.

Anxiety, mental stress, depression must be minimized and regulated because they decrease our immunity and predispose mental function deterioration. For our own good and that of others, we must be practical and solve conflicts in the best way. Remember that there is somatization or transformation of psychological symptoms or negative emotions into physical symptoms, simulating any disease.

We will delay aging as much as possible with these basic recommendations, reducing drug consumption and disease onset. The goal is not just to live as long as possible, but to live a longer, healthier, and happier life.

Being forever young is everyone's dream, and even more so with women. Every woman wants to maintain the same glam, beauty, poise, elegance, and grace they had in their twenties throughout their lifetime. However, nature has always had different plans for all of us.

Most women tend to recede and experience some changes in their bodies, particularly at age 40, which tends to mark a turning point for most women. At 40, our body chemistry begins to alter, our mood changes, and our weight is also affected. In this chapter we seek to discuss those changes and the reasons for them and in this chapter, we also look at hormonal alterations that begin to affect women after 40 and how best to be prepared for it and deal with it.

Just like in every other stage, this transitional stage comes with its challenges. Every woman must brace up and learn how to deal with this stage to get the best out of their lives. The midlife age is often triggered at the age of 40 in most women, where psychological, emotional, and physical changes begin to occur in the female body. Although these changes are things you are not likely used to, you must learn to understand them, embrace them and make the most of them to ensure that you will get the best out of the years ahead. At age 40, most women battle with a strong identity problem as they are no longer young, but neither are they old. Sometimes you might still feel young and try to do the things you used to do and consider it as normal as before. At other times, the body would reject what you want to do due to the changes occurring within it, making your body seem older.

Often, some drastic and noticeable changes begin to occur at age 40 due to hormonal changes as a result of the body beginning to prepare itself for menopause. However, many have argued that age 40 is relatively too low for women to experience menopause.

However, menopause does ever more frequently exist at this age, along with many of its complications. More women than ever are experiencing perimenopausal or menopausal symptoms and complications arising from these conditions in their early 40's and sometimes even earlier. These complications are a result of hormonal imbalance, which occurs when there are excess or inadequate hormones in the bloodstream. Menopause and perimenopause are significant events that alter the body's hormonal balance, resulting in great changes in the body.

What Are Hormones?

Hormones are biochemical substances generated by the glands in the body through the endocrine system. Hormones migrate through the bloodstream to tissues and organs, giving them messages that tell the organs what to do and dictate how they perform.

Hormones are essential in keeping the balance in most processes in the body as they affect metabolism, appetite, heart rate, sleep patterns, reproductive cycle, rate of growth, stress, mood, body temperature. Examples of hormones that affect both men and women are insulin, steroids, adrenaline, and some other hormones that induce growth.

Some other hormones are peculiar to women alone and are part of the major factors that influence the process of menopause, such as estrogen and progesterone.

Causes of Hormonal Imbalance in Women

Hormonal imbalance occurs at significant stages in the lives of women due to alterations in their body chemistry at these stages. Women are prone to have a hormonal imbalance at stages such as puberty, menstruation, pregnancy, childbirth, and breastfeeding. Women who are also in their mid - life span experience perimenopause, menopause, and post menopause.

As a result of these stages, in female development, women have a higher chance of developing hormonal imbalance than men due to the different endocrine and cycles they possess. Mostly mid- life span women start to suffer from changes to their hormonal balance as a result of perimenopausal or menopausal symptoms when they are around (before or after) 40.

What Are Perimenopause and Menopause?

Perimenopause

Perimenopause implies menopause. It is simply the time when your body begins to transition towards menopause and notes the end of your reproductive years. So, in an effort to put things into perspective, perimenopause is sometimes referred to as pre-menopause or menopausal transition. Although it occurs at different ages for women, the range at which it occurs tends to stay fairly constant. However, for some women it can occur in their mid-thirties. Most usually, however, it occurs in their forties and occasionally in the early '50s.

During the perimenopausal stage, the major hormone, in the female body, estrogen, starts to suffer random rises and falls in its levels and the menopausal cycles can also increase or decrease because of the irregular release of eggs from the ovaries. During this period, menstruation can be extremely irregular and uncertain.

However, after this period and if you have gone through 12months without a menstruation cycle, this means you have gone through the perimenopausal stage, and you are now into the menopausal period.

Menopause

Menopause is simply defined as the period where the ovaries no longer produce eggs, thus resulting in infertility and the stoppage of menstruation.

Changes That Women Experience During Perimenopause and Menopause

Reduced rate of metabolism.

As we age, the rate at which our body produces energy begins to reduce. This means that the physical activities you engaged in before would now become difficult in which to participate. Even if you are able to perform these activities, the level of calories burnt during the exercises becomes much reduced. This leads to a decrease in the amount of energy produced and makes the unburnt calories turn into fat. In order, to deal with this change, some simple steps need to be taken. Simple might, however, not mean easy as you would be stretched and would have to commit to certain lifestyle changes.

This change in lifestyle means you would reduce your calorie intake and step up in your normal exercise, which would enable you to maintain your body weight and retain the energy level of your younger self. The rationale behind this lifestyle change is clear. The reduced calorie intake would reduce the number of unused calories, while an increase in your normal exercise would help burn the number of unused calories left. Doing this while in your mid-life span would also help your body conditioning as they form the necessary habits needed to keep you in shape.

Ultimately, healthy lifestyles to enhance metabolism will, in the long run, enhance your longevity.

Hair Loss or Falling Out

At the age of 40, There is a lot going on in your body on a varied number of fronts and that is why you would hardly notice or hear people discuss hair loss at this stage. However, the loss of hair at this stage is more widely spread than you can possibly imagine. For most women, it starts at the age of 40; for a few, it starts in their early '30s.

According to one expert with Women's Health Associates, in the Department of Medicine, at the Massachusetts General Hospital in Boston, *"The hair loss occurs everywhere. This means that you potentially have to shave less of your pubic hair, depending on how you feel about it. There are a lot of effective options for your head. If you are worried about what happens to your overall body, it is not an overnight change, as once it has begun it progresses pretty slowly for several years ".*

Although it is a common occurrence, nevertheless it is important to know why it occurs. Our estrogen level's play a crucial role in the hair growth of women. So, it is no wonder why the hair of women thins out as they approach menopause; this is because the estrogen level of women decreases markedly as they approach this period resulting in hair loss.

There are a number of ways to help deal with this situation, you can reduce the number of times you wash your hair to reduce its falling out, as the natural oils produced by your scalp would help lubricate your hair. You could also use a natural shampoo and conditioner and reduce the number of styling tools that make use of heat, as well as reduce the number of products and processes, including coloring that you expose your hair to.

For menopausal victims experiencing hair loss, you may also wish to consult your Healthcare provider as there may be an option to help stimulate hair growth available.

Loss of Bladder Control.

Once again, estrogen is the causative hormone in this regard. Asides from this, Strains on the bladder as a result of childbearing and other activities can accumulate and have a compound effect on the strength of the muscles of the bladder as its production decreases with the advent of perimenopause.

The reduction in the production of estrogen simply means that there will be a reduction in the strength of the muscles that support the bladder and the urethra. These weakened muscles imply that you cannot cough, sneeze or actively laugh as you please. As serious as this might seem, there are solutions to help you deal with this embarrassing anomaly. These solutions would help you laugh, cough, and sneeze as you please. One of these solutions is taking off a few pounds while reducing pressure on your bladder, others are reducing the amount of alcohol and caffeinated drinks you consume. Kegel exercises would also help strengthen and rebuild the weakened muscles of the bladder and urethra. Should any of these methods fail in helping you eventually deal with the situation, your OBS-GYN doctor will help treat you by offering efficient medical options.

Loss of Memory

Have you ever stood in front of the wardrobe and wondered what you were doing there? It happens to the best of us. Your brain goes AWOL or begins losing some of its functions. This is a common occurrence among women, especially for those within the perimenopause, menopausal and post menopause stage. This unavoidable incident is also the fault of the ovaries because of their inability to produce the necessary amount of estrogen in your mid-life span.

Generally, women possess estrogen receptors in two parts of the brain, which control the brain's memory. The first part of the brain is referred to as the hippocampus, which is the memory center of the brain, while the second part is referred to as the prefrontal cortex, which arranges information and affects how we remember it. Estrogen also enhances the level of acetylcholine which is a neurotransmitter that aids the formation of new memories.

Whenever there is an inadequate amount of estrogen, which alters the structure of the brain negatively in those parts of the brain, again, don't worry, this consequence can be managed. This is because the functionality of your brain depends largely on the amount of oxygen given to it by the bloodstream. This implies that whatever is good for your brain is good for your heart. Therefore, the way to deal with this is to engage in activities that boost the performance of the heart, which would help the overall functionality of the brain.

Examples of such activities are intense exercise, a healthy diet plan, and a robust stress Management program. Also, you should engage in activities that help boost and exercise the brain. Activities such as crossword puzzles, reading complicated and comprehensive books, and other similar brain exercises will boost your overall brain functionality. Interestingly, the memory loss isn't permanent as it would fade off along with the menopause stage. You might consider helping your brain with estrogen therapy which some find helpful; however, the brain itself eventually adjusts itself to a lower level of estrogen and works fine with it. Besides, a period of temporary memory loss isn't enough to excuse for anyone to engage in hormone therapy which can carry a risk of breast cancer, heart disease, or stroke. It is always best to consult your Healthcare provider or medical professional for advice in this situation.

Urinary Problems

Generally, problems associated with the urinary system increase as you get older and become pronounced, particularly at the age of 40. Lauren Streicher, M.D., who is a director at the Center for Sexual Medicine and Menopause at Northwestern University's Feinberg School of Medicine, stated that estrogen is a strong hormone that helps protect the urinary path of the body against bacteria that often result in urinary tract infections. As women get older and approach 40, they become more likely to get infected because of the reduction in the amount of estrogen produced by the ovaries. This simple process has resulted in a lot of urinary tract infections in perimenopausal and menopausal women and has resulted in the ovaries of patients suffering this shut down completely. Often these, urinary tract infections are treated by antibiotics which take the place of or supplements the inadequate estrogen and fight off the bacteria that help protect the urinary tract. In fact, with the proper administration of these antibiotics, symptoms of urinary tract infections are often likely to disappear in two days.

With Antibiotics, it is important to finish the dosage course, Oftentimes, in the middle in the middle of the dosage course, you might start feeling better and might be tempted to stop using the drug altogether. Despite this, you must persist and keep using the drug until the dosage course is complete to prevent the urinary tract infection from returning.

Fluctuating and Unpredictable Menstrual Cycle in Your 40's

Of course, it goes without saying that before entering the postmenopausal stage, your menstruation must have ceased completely for at least a period of twelve months, however in the period that precedes this, which is the perimenopausal stage and the menopausal stage itself, menstruation fluctuates and can be wildly unpredictable. The reason for this is not far-fetched, as estrogen is largely responsible for the release of eggs from the ovaries, which cause menstruation. Therefore, the inadequate and unpredictable production of estrogen always results in fluctuating menstrual cycles. Sometimes some periods are close; other times, they are months apart. In some cycles, there might be a case of you having flowed heavier than normal, and some months, where there is no flow at all. The approach to ameliorating the effect of fluctuating menstrual cycles is often by the use of oral contraceptives or hormones releasing IUDs which are often prescribed under the auspices of your Healthcare provider, If the irregularities of your menstrual cycle persist, you should definitely see your OB-GYN doctor.

Vaginal Dryness

One of the most common problems associated with age which occurs in middle ages (40), is vaginal dryness. A renowned doctor, Doctor Ali Badi, was asked about sex and the dryness of the vaginal on a television show run by doctors, and she stated that " low and inadequate hormones levels make the vaginal wall thick and thin. Therefore, vaginal sexual activities are extremely important in helping to initiate blood flow to the vagina and to maintain the firmness of its muscle and to maintain its elasticity as well as its length". To deal with vaginal dryness, you could visit a pharmacy to buy an over counter vaginal lubricant or consult your doctor to prescribe a drug or vaginal hormone cream.

Loss of Estrogen

Estrogen is the major hormone in women, which is responsible for a variety of factors and has driven the symptoms of menopause while trying to cope with the low level of estrogen. Do you think hormone therapy is a plausible solution to solve all the problems?

Throughout this chapter, the relationship between the ovaries and the estrogen hormone has been pronounced, as these organs are responsible for the low production of estrogen. In fact, the inefficiency of the ovaries starts at around 40, precisely during the perimenopausal period, and stretches through the entire menopausal stage. With any disadvantages and discomfort that the inadequacy of estrogen brings, why not replace the insufficient amount through hormone therapy?

Generally, traditional hormone therapy increases the chances of breast cancer, heart diseases, and stroke. Therefore, completely outweighing the minor discomfort that many women in their 40's face. In the event, that traditional therapy is compulsory, it must be carried out by a specialist physician, who is normally a gynecologist.

However, there is a chance to still get the effect the traditional hormonal therapy gives through the application of the localized estrogen. Localized estrogen is applied as a topical cream, which delivers a lower level of estrogen compared to traditional hormonal therapy and carries less of the risk that the latter carries. The hormone from the local estrogen is assimilated directly into the bloodstream, hence it has a lesser chance of affecting the rest of the body.

In any event, it is important to consult your doctor (gynecologist) to know if the local estrogen is an option suitable for you. Generally, a change in lifestyle and the use of natural supplements are vital in the adequate production of estrogen and in guaranteeing the overall wellness of the body, even in the midst of symptoms of menopause and perimenopause.

Hot Flashes and Sleep Issues

Insomnia is a big problem for anyone as the body needs to rest after the day's work. Imagine a 40-year-old dealing with hair loss, irregular periods, vaginal problems, which are compounded with sleepless nights. That would certainly prove to be a handful and a lot for people to handle. Insomnia is a common occurrence for people in their perimenopausal stage as they experience hot flashes during their sleep.

This is a result of a variation in the intensity, length, and frequency of hot flashes. Sleepless nights are caused by hot flashes or night sweats. In fact, the body is used to them such that your sleep pattern might not be predictable without them. To deal with this, you could get a white sound noise machine that would help stabilize the frequency and intensity of sound within the room by making calm, soothing sounds that would relax you and help you to sleep better.

Mood Swings

The menopausal stage is an extremely challenging stage for anyone as you would have to deal with a whole lot of things as you pass through a stage that you have never been through before. When going through unpleasant situations or any form of discomfort, for that matter, you are likely to feel agitated and be really touchy, reacting like this is normal and understandable, as you are going through a whole lot of unpleasantness because of the inadequacy of estrogen in your body.

It would certainly come as no surprise, if your behavior alters and you react to things differently instead of the way you normally do. Mood swings and cases of depression and sadness often occur during perimenopause. Of all the symptoms of menopause and perimenopause, one symptom capable of causing mood swings is a disruption of your sleep pattern, which is often caused by hot flashes. Furthermore, changes in your mood might also be caused by factors not associated with hormonal sufficiency.

Decreasing Fertility

This is one of the most pronounced consequences of menopause as it highlights the end of your productive years, which is highlighted with the end of menstruation. Menstruation simply works through ovulation which is the release of eggs which is even shredded if it is not fertilized by a sperm. The regular release of the eggs shows fertility and your ability to get pregnant.

And since ovulation becomes irregular and unpredictable, menstruation fluctuates, your ability to give birth or get pregnant also decreases. Nevertheless, as long as, you are still having your period or menstruation, you can get pregnant. This is because your period shows that an egg, even though it is unfertilized in the event of this, is characterized by fluctuating periods. It is best to use contraceptives and other birth control methods to prevent pregnancy and not to rely on the fluctuating ovulation cycle. You are only sure that you require no contraceptives while trying to prevent pregnancy only when you have not experienced your period for 12 consecutive months

Alterations in Sexual Function.

Several changes occur in the perimenopausal stage and in the menopausal stage. One major change is the alteration in your sex drive. Normally, if you had a strong sex drive prior to your menopausal stage, it can still be maintained throughout the entirety of the menopausal stage and even more than the menopausal stage. This is because, while oftentimes, the alterations are drastic, sometimes they are not.

Weakness in The Bones and Loss of Bone Density.

The estrogen hormone certainly affects a number of factors, including the strength and density of your bones. With reduced estrogen levels, you are likely to lose more bone mass than you can replace. This fact increases your chances of having osteoporosis which is a disease that results in having fragile bones.

Alteration in Cholesterol Levels

Most people think cholesterol results in obesity, and it's not necessarily good for the body. However, there are good cholesterols that are vital to the overall performance of your body. There are two types of cholesterol: the low density of lipoprotein, which is the bad cholesterol, and the high-density lipoprotein, which is the good cholesterol. Bad cholesterol, which is the low-density lipoprotein (LDL), increases the chances of heart diseases, while the good cholesterol high-density lipoprotein (HDL) reduces the risk of heart diseases.

Your estrogen levels affect the composition and concentration of both proteins in a disadvantageous way to the body. The reduced estrogen causes an increase in the Low-density of Lipoprotein (bad cholesterol) and causes a decrease in the High-density Lipoprotein (Good cholesterol), thereby increasing the risk of heart diseases in the body.

Factors Affecting the Emergence and Intensity of These Symptoms

Menopausal stages come with complications as well as symptoms. However, what accounts for its intensity and its early emergence varies considerably. Here are some factors that affect its intensity and its early emergence.

Smoking

According to research, estrogen levels have been observed to decrease two years earlier in those who smoke as opposed to those who do not. This implies that menopause can occur at least a year or two years earlier in female smokers than in their non-smoking counterparts.

Heredity

Heredity also plays an important role in predicting the health of an individual and how to cope and manage it. The body composition of parents tends to be transferred through genes to their offspring. Therefore, if there is a history of early menopausal experiences in your family, there is a great chance that you would experience it as well.

Treatment of Cancer

The treatment of cancer can often be harsh and intense thereby, causing a lot of side effects within the body and one of these side effects is the early emergence of menopause. Therefore, treating cancer by means such as chemotherapy or pelvic radiation is likely to result in early menopause.

Hysterectomy

Normally hysterectomy is the removal of the uterus without the ovaries, which does not result in menopause. You might not experience your periods anymore. Nevertheless, your ovaries still produce estrogen, and it's a major cause of menopause. Therefore, this kind of surgery might cause menopause to appear a lot earlier than expected.

Why Intermittent Fasting Is Key to Dealing with Menopause

Intermittent fasting is a method of eating that is characterized by a period of fasting mixed with periods of eating. Studies have shown that intermittent fasting can help deal expedite weight loss, especially in men. Intermittent fasting basically works due to the reduced number of calories you consume. This pattern of eating encourages weight loss because of the way the metabolism works within the body and because the body does not use all the calories it consumes.

Therefore, the excess ones are stored as fat as the body fat. Anytime you fast, the calories store as fat to compensate for the shortage of calories. This process helps burn fat really fast. Intermittent fasting is similar to but quite different from the ketogenic diet, while intermittent fasting makes use of actual fasting while ketogenic diet basically watches what you eat. A ketogenic diet is the consumption of a low carbohydrate, high-fat diet. Sometimes, intermittent fasting is best combined with a ketogenic diet to get the desired result. Some might fast twice a week for outright 24hours while some fast alternatively for sixteen hours throughout the week. Furthermore, during these fasting periods it is advised to avoid processed food as it will not help you to get back in shape or help to accelerate your weight loss.

How Can Intermittent Fasting Help Deal with Pre - Menopausal Weight Gain?

Intermittent Fasting undoubtedly reduces the number of calories you consume. As we all know, being in calorie deficient is vital to achieving weight loss. Generally, Menopausal women have poor sleep patterns and age due to series of hormonal changes. Therefore, Intermittent Fasting will reduce the number of calories and help them lose weight. In the same vein, weight control will also be effectively managed through the process. Furthermore, the Keto diet will help intermittent fasting and prevent you from breaking it with processed, unwholesome foods.

Here are some tips to help with intermittent fasting and help you deal with menopause:

Start Slowly with Short Fasting Periods

It is best to start slowly in a journey and finish strong; one of the ways to ensure that you go the distance in a journey, is to conserve energy and release when it is needed. You could also start with the length of the fasting period you are comfortable with and build it up from there.

Don't Be Too Rigid with Your Calorie Intake

Sometimes, when you feel like consuming more, it is actually because your body is telling you that it needs more calories since most of the biological changes fluctuate. Therefore, it is best not to be rigid and try to listen to your inner self before acting. It will not hurt to take in a few extra calories when you feel you need it.

Take A Lot of Water

Taking a lot of water does not break your fast in any way; rather, it helps you stay hydrated and allows you to go for the Long haul. You could also take unsweetened coffee, which will help contain hunger for a while.

Find A New Hobby

Intermittent Fasting can take a long time to master and is a marathon. Therefore, to stick with a marathon, you must be able to stay till the end. To do this, it may find a hobby that will help you pass the time and endure during the fast.

Seek the Help of a Professional

You can always seek the help of a nutritionist to help you get the best nutrition plan, Since Intermittent Fasting is a continuous regime. Therefore, it is best to find the version for you, to fit into your lifestyle and to help you lose weight.

Weakness in The Bones and the Loss of Bone Density

As previously mentioned, the estrogen hormone certainly affects a number of factors, including the strength and Density of your bones; with reduced estrogen levels, you are likely to lose more bone mass than you can replace. This fact increases your chances of having osteoporosis which is a disease that results in having fragile bones

CHAPTER THIRTEEN

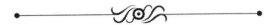

INTERMITTENT FASTING AND EXERCISE

Intermittent Fasting is widely known for its health benefits. The same can be said for exercise. But what about combining intermittent fasting with exercise?

The term "fast cardio" is a contentious topic that has divided the health and fitness community for years. People have debated about this a lot and sometimes tend to overlook the nuances of combining intermittent fasting with exercise.

Starving yourself and spending hours on the treadmill do not fit the definition of a healthy person, but what about more moderate methods?

Is Fasting Exercise Safe or A good idea?

Scientists, researchers, and trainers are still debating the benefits of fasting exercise for weight loss. And scientific studies have produced conflicting results in this area, so the Jury is still out on this issue. The good news is that most people can safely exercise on an empty stomach.

Without a doubt, humans have always exercised on an empty stomach; our bodies can survive and thrive on long fasts, and our forefathers were definitely not couch potatoes.

Now that we have that important question out of the way, what are the drawbacks to combining exercise and intermittent fasting?

Disadvantages of Exercising on An Empty Stomach

The following are some of the potential drawbacks of exercising on an empty stomach:

- Combining the two practices can be difficult for people who are new to fasting or exercising. (When you are "hungry," you may eat too much too soon.)

- If you are already slim, exercising on an empty stomach can cause you to lose weight you may not want to.

Fasting does not improve acute exercise performance, so you should avoid competing or training hard during long fasts. However, as with any health or fitness topic, context is key, when weighing the benefits and drawbacks of fasting exercise. If in doubt, always consult a professional for advice.

But first, let us examine the health advantages of exercising while fasting!

Potential Health Benefits of Fasting and Exercise

- Increased fat oxidation

- Improved autophagy

- It helps regulate insulin sensitivity and blood sugar levels

- Greater metabolic flexibility (the ability to switch between carbohydrates and fat for fuel)

- Higher levels of human growth hormone (HGH)

- Aerobic exercise can help manage appetite and cravings, making it easier to fast

- It May help preserve muscle mass

- Improved aerobic condition

How the Benefits Work

The advantages of exercising on an empty stomach can be divided into three categories: metabolic, hormonal, and fitness benefits.

When you fast, your body switches from an anabolic to a catabolic state (energy storage and tissue building) (using stored energy and breaking down larger molecules into simpler molecules). While neither anabolism nor catabolism is inherently good or bad, our bodies function best when the two are balanced. As a result, intermittent fasting has considerable benefits over the practice of eating three meals a day, every day.

Essentially, the metabolic benefits of fasting translate into long-term health benefits due to effects like increased fat utilization and support for autophagy (the process of damaged cells being cleaned up by the body). Similarly, your body must use the available energy to cover physical activity's metabolic costs when you exercise. Your body can use the calories from the foods you just ate if you train in the fed state.

However, exercising on an empty stomach increases the demand for stored energy, enhancing your fasting period's metabolic benefits even further. Fasting and exercise, for example, improve insulin sensitivity and your body's ability to switch between carbohydrates and fat as a fuel source, which can benefit your overall health.

Beneficial hormonal changes include higher HGH levels and lower hunger hormones and the practice of exercising on an empty stomach can also improve your fitness results and spare lean muscle tissue during exercise because fasting or avoiding carbohydrates improves fat oxidation (fat burning), synonymous with improved aerobic fitness.

The Best Types of Exercise During Intermittent Fasting

Before embarking on any exercise program, be sure you seek advice from your medical professional.

- **Walking**

- Brisk walking for 30 minutes or more every day can help you avoid disease, maintain a healthy weight, and support your brain health as you age. Walking is also a good option if you are new to fasting for the following reasons:

- It is doable for people of all fitness levels, without the need for specialized skills

- It's free, without sports equipment

- The risk of injury is low

- This results in better fat oxidation

If you do not know where to start exercising on an empty stomach, start by walking. As you become more experienced, you can try other types of activities.

- **Low-Intensity Cardio (LISS)**

Low-intensity steady-state cardio (LISS) burns the most fat of any type of exercise while also improving aerobic fitness and heart health. LISS's fat oxidation, similar to walking, makes it an excellent choice for enhancing the benefits of fasting.

If you do not like running, there is good news: you can do anything else that keeps your heart rate in the fat-burning zone, such as biking, hiking, or any other steady-state activity (around 60-80 percent of your heart rate: heart rate maximum).

If you do not have a heart rate monitor, simply aim for an exercise intensity that allows you to speak in full sentences. If your goal is to improve your health and wellness, try 30-60 minutes of LISS on an empty stomach. For endurance athletes, longer durations may be appropriate.

- **Low-Intensity Interval Training (LIIT)**

LIIT (low-intensity interval training) is a type of exercise that is similar to LISS cardio in terms of intensity. LIIT, on the other hand, combines faster and slower intervals.

Cycling at a faster and slower pace, running and walking, or any other fast-slow (or hard-easy) combination are all popular LIIT options. For LIIT, some people also use circuit training. LIIT is an excellent choice for your fasting periods due to its low intensity. It is also a fun way to add variety to your workout if you are tired of walking and steady-state cardio.

Try a 1-to-5-minute fast interval followed by a 1-to-10-minute slower interval. Repeat for a total of 20 to 60 minutes, ensuring that you stay in the fat-burning zone throughout.

- **High-Intensity Interval Training (HIIT)**

HIIT (High-Intensity Interval Training) is like LIIT, but it is done at a higher intensity level. While high-intensity interval training (HIIT) is popular in the fitness world right now, it may not be the best option for some people who are fasting. This is why: High-intensity workouts are glycolytic, which means they use glucose (sugar) as a source of energy.

You are more likely to experience an unpleasant "crash" if you do glycolytic training on an empty stomach, especially if your muscles are already depleted of glycogen stores (stored glucose).

Furthermore, intense exercise promotes amino acid oxidation, leading to a loss of fasting muscle mass.

- **Resistance training and metabolic conditioning ("Metcon")**

Some people lift weights or do metabolic conditioning workouts (such as CrossFit) on an empty stomach, but this is not the best approach for everyone. An intense exercise that uses glucose for fuel is more difficult to maintain on an empty stomach, as we have just seen described above.

Furthermore, it has been proven that eating a pre-workout meal improves this type of performance. You will get better results in the fed state, especially if your goal is muscle gain because your weightlifting results are dependent on your level of performance.

The bottom line: If you are serious about strength training, you need to eat well before and after your workouts. Make the necessary adjustments to your sessions and you will notice the difference.

How to Exercise Optimally While You Are Fasting

- ## 16/8 and related forms of intermittent fasting

The best time to exercise on an empty stomach if you are on an 8/16 or similar fasting regimen with a set daily meal window is in the morning. According to some studies, exercising first thing in the morning on an empty stomach increases fat oxidation for at least 24 hours, potentially enhancing the benefits of your fasting period.

However, you can of course exercise at any time during your fasting period, so do not worry if you cannot get to the gym in the morning. If you prefer to eat early in the morning and fast later, make sure you do your cardio on an empty stomach at least 6 hours after your last meal. The majority of your last meal is in your small intestine after 6-8 hours, and it takes 5-6 hours for your body to empty after a meal.

Brisk walking, LISS, or LIIT are the best exercise options for your fasting periods, as we have seen before. If you want to incorporate HIIT, resistance training, or metcon workouts, you should schedule them after you have eaten at least one meal.

- ## Extended fasts (24 hours and more)

You can still include fasting exercise if your fasting strategy includes more than 24 hours of fasting. Early in the fast, you can use LISS and LIIT to improve fat oxidation and autophagy, but do not push yourself too hard or for too long until you have tried them a few times. Since your fast will last longer than 24 hours, brisk walking is the safest option, at least at first.

You may be able to use LISS and LIIT in your extended fasts once you have gained more experience, but it is best to gradually test your limits over several fasts.

Finally, eat 1 to 2 meals (preferably with moderate or high carbohydrates) after a long period of fasting before engaging in resistance training, metabolic conditioning, competition, or other performance-based activities.

Whether you combine fasting and exercise or not, both are extremely beneficial. Because of the synergy, exercising on an empty stomach can improve the health benefits of both practices.

However, if you are new to fasting or do not exercise regularly, you should consult your Medical professional first. You are probably fasting too long or training too hard if you feel weak, tired, or hungry. Make sure that you allow your body to adjust to fat burning, so be patient and in the meantime, combine brisk walking with shorter fasting periods.

CHAPTER FOURTEEN

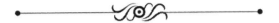

INTERMITTENT FAST AND HEALTH

Studies on the potential benefits of fasting have emerged in recent years, particularly since the 2016 Nobel Prize was awarded to the Japanese Yoshinori Ohsumi medical team, who discovered the health benefits of the metabolic process called autophagy.

It is a method by which the body can eliminate aberrant structures so that altered or tumor cells, viruses, bacteria, and other structures are simply "engulfed" by lysosomes, macrophages, and other immune system-derived processes that occur mainly in periods of fasting. It has been observed that autophagy occurs in the body after approximately 12 hours of fasting due to the activation of the AMPK metabolic pathway when glucose and insulin are at low levels.

Metabolic Syndrome

Without a doubt, both metabolic syndrome and all associated processes can be improved thanks to fasting. For example:

- Blood glucose and insulin fasting.

- HDL lipoprotein boost.

- Reduced visceral fat and lower triglycerides.

- Blood pressure control.

- Blood coagulation improvement and thrombosis and cardiovascular disease prevention.

- Development of the predisposition of metabolic syndrome-associated benign and malignant tumors.

Some studies influence different cholesterol fractions on the positive effect of fasting so that LDL appears to decrease and HDL increases.

Intermittent Fasting and Blood Pressure

Although there are no official trails or studies in which increases in blood pressure have been shown in intermittent fasting, we find that patients who have been consuming, or gradually decreasing calories for several days have displayed a drop in blood pressure. Up to 80% of subjects experience a significant drop in blood pressure from 3 or 4 days of fasting.

We must bear in mind that when a person fasts, insulin levels tend to decrease because we know that insulin is pro-inflammatory. It increases sodium retention and helps to produce fluid retention in the body, which also allows fasting and blood pressure to decrease.

Fasting and Weight Loss

It should be remembered that one of the benefits of trying to limit the number of calories to 8-10 hours is that people usually end up consuming less, and the studies conducted by Varady Et. Al in 2013 found that for 12 weeks, the correlation between a group of people who ate food for many hours and another group who practiced intermittent fasting resulted in an average reduction of 5.2 kg between the second of the listed groups after a few weeks. A fat reduction of 3.6 kg had also been observed, which is explained by the fact that there are more hours of low insulin levels when fasting, promoting metabolic activation associated with fat loss.

Some athletes are afraid that when fasting, results in a loss of muscle mass caused by proteolysis. However, numerous studies have been conducted in which the amount of nitrogen in urea (a good indicator of proteolysis) has been tested, concluding that it does not increase until 60 hours of fasting, so there should be no need for concern about the loss of muscle mass.

An interesting fact demonstrated by the scientist is that when undergoing an obese population nucleus study, both groups lose the same amount of weight relative to another group that performs fasting. However, those who practiced intermittent fasting decreased more kilos associated with fat mass (90%) than fat-free mass (10%). The group which performed a continuous caloric restriction lost 75% of weight in fat mass and up to 25% of fat-free mass, which means greater muscle mass loss and appeared to achieve a lower basal metabolic rate after a few weeks (as opposed to those that perform intermittent fasting).

People who make an ongoing caloric restriction have more problems with increased appetite, heart output, thyroid-level hormonal imbalances, growth hormone, glucagon, adrenaline, testosterone, etc. This does not happen, and even some parameters improve in people accustomed to fasting. We also know that in subjects who perform fasting levels of leptin, ghrelin or adiponectin, tend to be much more regulated, which means that appetite and satiety balance are more controlled because these hormones are directly responsible for these sensations.

Inflammation and Intermittent Fasting

When looking at people fasting in Ramadan. Modulation and enhancement of inflammation-related biomarkers (such as C-reactive protein, Interleukin 6, or Alfa tumor necrosis factor) were observed. People who made Ramadan appeared to lower the body's levels of inflammation. We also find that the AMPK enzyme pathway activity increases after 12 hours of fasting, consistent with autophagy and immune system regulation with reduced body inflammation.

Biorhythms and Fasting

Intermittent fasting imposes a daily pattern on the Body's food consumption, which makes the person able to better adapt to the biological cycles of day/night. The Body consumes food for 8 hours a day, and in effect, states that this intake will not be continued during the following 16 hours. The body recognizes eating during daylight hours, and the hypothalamus receives an activation that has an extremely positive effect on the rest of the glandular, hormonal, and immunological function.

The digestive system is one of the systems that most benefits from regulating circadian rhythms as many of its functions are closely related to these rhythms. For example, stomach emptying, blood flow at mesenteric vessel level (which must be higher during the day than at night), as well as all metabolic functions associated with the pancreas, gallbladder, or liver that allows all digestive, metabolic functions to be active during the day and slows them down at night.

Likewise, it has been shown that if at night food is ingested, the quality and duration of sleep are usually affected, in addition to the fact that insulin resistance and an alteration in the release of growth hormone and different neurohormones are linked to tissue recovery and repair.

Fasting and Brain Function

Fasting has been shown to have a beneficial effect on the brain's level of neuronal activity. First of all, by recomposing the organism (Body) in the day/night cycles, this provides an incredibly positive hormonal modulation and causes the dopamine levels to be high in the morning (which allows the person to be regularly active). The serotonin levels will remain high at night, which will be beneficial to the rest. By having the lowest levels of fasting insulin, a greater release of growth hormone and more neurotrophic factors derived from the brain are permitted at night, which makes the person more neuroplastic and can much better prevent neurodegenerative pathologies like Alzheimer's, Parkinson's, or multiple sclerosis. The body releases neuglucogenic hormones (growth hormone, glucagon, cortisol, adrenaline) throughout the day by having a lower fasting blood glucose and insulin. On the contrary, people with high glucose and insulin fasting levels usually suffer from a slowdown in mental dullness and thinking.

Fasting and Digestive System

Fasting methods have been used since ancient times to treat all sorts of intestinal problems such as gastritis, esophagitis, gastroesofático reflux, irritable bowel syndrome, dyspepsia, severe fermentation, etc. In the animal kingdom, we will find a curious fact that when there is a stagnant food bolus, they need to digest or have an issue with the stomach, the animals fast from solid food and drink only water. This is a physiological mechanism that allows the return

116

to equilibrium of all intestinal functions during the hours when no work is done in the digestive system.

Intermittent fasting favors that the levels of hydration in the stomach mucosa, the release of hydrochloric acid by the stomach, or the release of enzymes and bile acids return to normal during the 14-16 hours the solid intake is not made. Similarly, we know that the intestinal flora continues to stabilize during fasting. The bacterial strains are balanced, causing some pathogenic strains not to proliferate excessively (e.g., Helicobacter pylori, candida, or other forms of intestinal pathogens). It has also been proven that there are clear benefits in fasting for ulcerative colitis, digestive systems, and irritable bowel syndrome.

Fasting and Cancer

More and more scientists are trying to help cancer patients aim to change the oncological metabolic process to complement traditional treatments (chemotherapy, radiotherapy, surgery). In recent years, studies have been reported in which, at the time of intermittent fasting in both animals and humans, the modulating effects at the stage of metabolism were observed. Several volunteers underwent a study in which the medical team discovered how glucose-insulin levels and, most importantly, the IGF-1 values (which is a potential oncological marker) were greatly improved by fasting cardiovascular risk indicators.

Intermittent Fast Confection

Is focused on having enough fasting hours from the last to the first intake of the next day, distributing amounts of glucose, insulin, inhibiting the mTOR's anabolic pathway, and activating the autophagic pathway of the AMPK. It has been noted that this starts to happen after 12 hours of fasting, although the ideal is to arrive between the last meal and the first intake of the next day until 14-16 hours of fasting.

The instructions to follow depend greatly on each person's schedules and customs, but the intermittent fasting rule, in general, suggests that after getting up, there must be 3-4 hours in which no food has been consumed, thereby increasing the glucose levels. Insulin and neuglucogenic hormones (adrenaline, norepinephrine, glucagon, growth hormone, cortisol) will be released, t4 to t3 conversion at a molecular level will be favored, and free testosterone bioavailability will be improved in the early morning hours. This will encourage the autophagic routes triggering at the start of the day and mobilize the accumulated fatty acids in the visceral fat adipocytes.

Upon getting up, ideally the first intake would be after 3-4 hours. Some people take the opportunity to do their first fasting training at this point, so it is done with low glucose and a lot of insulin sensitivity, which encourages a high-fat energy mobilization, with high lipolysis and induced thermogenesis because glucose levels are small when training starts. Others chose to go with one hour and a half or two hours before exercise is advised to make the first intake in other situations. In order, to extend the activation of the AMPK route, this first intake of nourishment should consist of protein and fat, particularly with medium-chain triglycerides found in good fats like coconut oil. In this way, the mitochondrial activity that works very efficiently from the medium-chain triglycerides will be remarkably high.

Following the general guidance, any carbohydrate intake should be done once the first practice is completed, thus breaking the AMPK route's function and activating the mTOR route linked to insulin receptor activation and hyperexpression of the body's proteins. Because of this super-compensation mechanism and improved insulin sensitivity in the previous 14-18 hours, the person can assimilate the carbohydrate much better at this stage and generate a more beneficial impact through insulin, enabling them to refill better glycogen activation routes intended for tissue formation and recovery.

Then we are going to have further meals before we hit about 8 hours of food intake that must contain glycemic index carbohydrates and proteins. What is important to note is that If a person wishes to practice intermittent fasting during even days of the week and there are days when he does not exercise, the ideal for health purposes and to maintain low insulin levels is to reduce the amount of carbohydrate during the non-exercise days and increase the amount of fat to have to ensure the elevated metabolic pathway of AMPK. It should also be noted that fasting would not be one of the best strategies in high-performance athletes or people who need to eat extremely high calorie levels throughout the day or those who are in the process of muscle hypertrophy because, in these situations, you need to consume extremely high calorie levels (especially carbohydrates) to have maximum glycogen levels, and this may cause problems at the intestinal level. Nevertheless, to boost hormonal levels and bowel functions, high-level athletes may benefit from one or two days a week of fasting.

Intermittent Fasting is a proven technique of weight loss that involves interposing fasting periods with feeding periods. Not only "mere mortals" use this routine: some athletes also use this method to remove fats that hinder their bodies.

Thanks to its simplicity and its proven success ratio, this type of diet is becoming extremely popular. The approach is simply to disrupt food consumption over a certain period.

It also forces the body to use its fat "reserves" to protect the biological unit. The body begins to lose weight slowly in this cycle of eating its reserves.

It certainly seems like a simple diet to follow through, but a lot of the specifics contained in this book will make all the difference to you, especially, if you want to understand how it works and practice intermittent fasting successfully to achieve the best results.

Who Cannot Do This?

Most people can perform this diet. However, certain sectors of the population cannot perform this kind of regime.

For example:

1. People who are below their weight

There is no need for these diets for people who are below their ideal weight for obvious reasons. For example, having a good notion of weight is sometimes hard and you may wish to consult your Healthcare provider for help with this and have them answer your questions from a medical perspective.

2. Pregnant and lactating

This diet is extremely dangerous for pregnant women as well as breastfeeding mothers. The main reason is that in both situations, the woman needs nutrients and proteins.

A sharp supply change can lead to weakness, hypoglycemia, and anemia. Not counting that the baby will suffer the effects of nutrient shortages. They also need enough nutrients and especially in the case of lactating women who need to produce breast milk. Breast milk is important for babies to develop healthily.

3. People with chronic diseases

Some medicines used to treat chronic diseases, such as diabetes or hypertension, cause metabolism changes and, eventually, lead to a picture of hypoglycemia.

For such phenomena, anyone who suffers from these diseases and wants to lose weight has most definitely to consult their Medical practitioner to see whether this kind of regime would be suitable for them and if so, it is also advisable to consult a nutritionist who will be responsible for directing the consumption of foods that cover basic needs.

4. Children and teenagers

While teenagers are commonly seen in these types of diets, these eating interruptions are dangerous, particularly during the growing phases. In childhood, carrying out these interruptions may cause problems with their development, and in the case of an adolescent's hormonal disorders.

It can cause serious health problems, both physical and psychological, in teenagers and adolescence knowing that they are in a very intense hormonal development stage. Also, it could cause issues in the psyche, the adolescent can develop severe eating disorders such as bulimia (strong and almost uncontrollable vomiting) and anorexia (the nearly schizophrenic notion of the constant need to lose weight at any cost).

5. Seniors

Over time, the body becomes much more fragile to changes. When there is a nutritional change, as in intermittent fasting, it has more potent effects on the body when it is older Because of these consequences, the elderly are generally much more sensitive to diseases related to the body and its biological system. Therefore, before embarking on a program of this time and you definitely need to consult your Healthcare provider and remember that medical follow-ups, both endocrinologist and nutritionist, are mandatory.

How to Use Intermittent Fasting Benefits to Better Your Life

There are many advantages of intermittent fasting that scientists have found in respect of reducing caloric intake for one cause or another. Intermittent fasting has been described in basic terms as some fifteen hours without eating. With this approach, the body will adjust several characteristics for the better.

The real question is not if fasting can help you or not, but more to the point, How it will help you and how often you should practice it.

This fasting style has been shown to lower blood pressure and increase levels of HDL. It can help greatly with diabetes management and will also help you lose weight. All these effects sound surprisingly good and can be achieved with the fasting of this type. Studies carried out on several different animal species show that limiting caloric intake increases their lives by 30 percent.

Human studies show it reduces blood pressure, blood sugar, and sensitivity to insulin. With these experiments, it has been shown that fasting could improve a human's life if performed for an extended period.

Cutting our calorie intake by 30 percent will achieve the same results, However, just doing this alone has been shown to cause depression and irritability. Fasting is an alternative method offered instead of simply cutting calories and it has demonstrated that it provides benefits without the side effects of stress or irritability.

Intermittent fasting is a great way of getting into better physical condition, living a longer, healthier life, and feeling better all the time.

Diet to Reduce Stress and Increase Happiness

There is a strong relationship between stress and our body. For example, muscle tension is a physical reflex reaction to stress; it is the body's way of protecting itself against danger. It may feel like a little ache or something tightening in the back of your neck or lower back as you type on the computer. Headaches are a close cousin. The relationship is so strong that it has its own term: Stress Headaches (also known as "tension pains").

Stress even causes digestive problems as it alters the concentration of acid in the stomach which can lead to inflammation, colic, diarrhea, constipation, irritable bowel syndrome, and even peptic ulcers. Stress disrupts the body's insulin production, leading to diabetes and even heart attacks or strokes. Healthy diets have been shown to prevent these damaging physical effects of stress and even reverse the aging process. Life is short, and optimizing your diet is an easy way to take control and maximize your well-being especially if you are a woman over 40.

Eating a healthy balanced diet is the key to health and wellbeing throughout our lives and furthermore if you are woman over 40 in a high-pressured Business environment, good nutrition will make a huge difference to your health and well-being and aid you to become a more effective leader. You owe it to yourself to properly feed your body and brain, so here are four steps to creating a successful eating plan for those in high stress and pressured work environments.

1. Give Priority to Breakfast

In a high- pressured Business environment, starting the day well is important, even more so for women over 40. In this kind of situation, you should get into the habit of eating breakfast. Skipping breakfast when you are under pressure can make it difficult to maintain stable blood sugar levels. What you give to your body at this time of day is also vitally important. Try to choose foods high in fiber like cereals, oatmeal, whole wheat bread, and fresh fruit. High-fiber foods digest more slowly and keep you satisfied, as well as jump-start your metabolism and stabilize your blood sugar levels, allowing you to focus and reduce your anxiety and stress.

As a leader, breakfast may be the most important meal of the day, but it does not just end there. Intermittent fasting for sugar control and weight loss can enhance your mind and the positively affect the relationships you have with your team. When you value the connection between your stomach and your mind, you get the most out of your day.

This gift, that is, life, is quite short and fleeting, Make the Most of It.

2. Limit your Consumption of Refined Sugars and Processed Foods

Certain foods are toxic to your brain. You should stay away from refined sugar. Try to avoid foods that are high in white sugar and high fructose corn syrup. And you should not give these foods to your team either, especially, if you want them to be set for success too.

Low-sugar diets have been shown to increase brain neurotrophic factor (BDNF), a peptide responsible for creating new neurons. This peptide makes neurons connect and combine, in addition to playing a fundamental role in neuroplasticity.

Try to avoid filling your kitchen with products high in sugar and foods with a high glycemic index, such as slices of bread, sweet drinks, and fast food. Much better try fruit and honey, (see also the list of Superfoods for Women over 40) Or better yet, go for a natural protein like soy that will help you build muscle. Refined sugars will always give you a quick energy boost, but you will soon feel like your blood sugar is on a roller coaster ride and most definitely not a fun one.

When sugar levels drop, your adrenal glands release stress hormones like cortisol. This will affect your performance as a leader. You will become more impatient and irritable in conversations, your relationships will suffer, and you will not make the correct decisions that your team needs.

3. Include Omega-Three Fatty Acids

Omega 3 fatty acids are gifts for any leader, and are especially important for women over 40, these deserve to be included in your diet. Nuts and seeds, including chia and flaxseed, and walnuts, are your best friends and partners. Nuts are known to protect the heart and contain antioxidants. Walnuts are a particularly healthy and a rich source of omega-three fatty acids that reduce the risk of heart attacks and bad cholesterol. Omega 3s help to stabilize adrenal hormones and prevent them from spiking, especially when you are under pressure, thus becoming a powerful antidote to stress.

4. Limit Your Intake of Caffeine and Alcohol

Craving caffeinated foods is natural. We all crave coffee, tea, soda, or chocolate, but it's important to recognize that these foods and drinks can affect our overall well-being. Caffeine stimulates the production of cortisol, the stress hormone. Having an occasional cup of coffee is fine but try to avoid it before bed because it can give you insomnia. You should also think about when and how to consume alcohol. Alcohol is a depressant and has a sedative effect that alters neurotransmitters in the brain. Having a couple of beers or a couple of glasses of wine after work may sound tempting but try not to overdo this habit because it could negatively affect your performance as a leader.

When you are stressed, it is easier to indulge in cravings and give in to impulses, often facilitating drug or alcohol use as a defense mechanism. In the long term, this can result in addictions. It is best to avoid these temptations when you are experiencing high levels of stress.

Your eating habits and the quality of the nutrition you are ingesting together with level of stress you handle, go hand in hand.

When you are stressed, it is natural to crave comfort foods like desserts, fast food, and alcohol, but these foods can be addictive and set you off on a dead-end spiral.

Fueling your body for success will reduce stress, improve your productivity, and strengthen your relationship with your team, so keep these four steps in mind to create a high-performance eating plan.

Tips to Start A Healthy Life

1. Learn something new every day. Healthy and successful people, regardless of their age, are eternal dreamers. They are well rounded and balanced individuals who work hard, play hard and think hard. They love to read, listen to audiobooks, and absorb as much knowledge as possible. They educate themselves on topics relevant to their business and their personal interests; they also seek knowledge of other types. They know that healthy and well-balanced behaviors have a positive impact on their lives.

2. Set goals and create systems to achieve them. Healthy successful people understand that knowledge without application is the fastest path to failure. They go beyond learning - they apply and share what they have learned. They realize that daily journeys and steps are the only way to achieve goals.

3. Spend your leisure time wisely. The average person spends three hours a day watching television. Don't be that kind of person.

1. To stay healthy, focus on the things that are important to you, take care of yourself and your family.

4. Make exercise a priority. A healthy body helps cultivate a healthy mind. An adult should exercise 2.5 hours a week or more with a variety of different types of exercise and intensity levels. Doing so, will help you relieve stress and get those endorphins flowing to help you to overcome your challenges.

2. 5.Try to eliminate or at least eat less junk food.

3. Think of food as fuel: The higher the quality of fuel you put in your tank, the better you will perform. Try to eat more real foods (that come from nature), instead of processed and fast food. Doing so will improve your energy level and mood, among other benefits.

4. 6. Get more sleep. Everyone will experience sleepless nights, early morning meetings, and last-minute deliveries. But a healthy person knows that sleep is essential to their success. it is important to find a consistent sleep routine and stick with it. Do not underestimate the power of a good nap to recharge your brain, either.

6. Create a balance in your life. Healthy successful people, treat their health as a lifestyle. Successful people adopt a healthy lifestyle: they work smart, both on a personal and professional level, they don't work aimlessly or continually anymore.

Golden Rules to Keep in Mind to Lose Weight

The experts are overwhelmingly clear: to lose weight successfully and maintain it in the long term, regardless of age; the key is, to follow a varied and balanced diet and accompany it with some physical exercise.

Do not forget these premises:

Balance and Moderation

Any weight loss plan aims to eat fewer calories than the body spends to create a caloric deficit.

Fundamental to Do Sports

Cardiovascular Exercises Such as fast walking, cycling, or running are the most effective at removing excess fat from the body.

Dieting Does Not Mean Starving

The real key is not in quantity but quality. You should know how to choose well and always opt for those foods with a lower caloric intake.

It's Not About Dieting, But About Changing Habits

It is useless for you to spend three months on a demanding and restrictive regimen if afterward, you will return to the same inadequate diet as always. If what you want is to lose weight and to maintain it in the long run, you should not view the diet as a special way of feeding during a specific period but more as a change of habits for a lifetime.

Compensation Law Applies

This is the most logical approach......

If you overspend on calories one day at lunch, you then try to eat a lighter dinner to compensate and thus not affect the total daily calories.

Dieting Does Not Mean Having to Give Up Meetings with Friends and Family

In most bars and restaurants, they offer light and healthy alternatives such as salads, vegetable dishes, fish, or grilled meats.

Enjoy What You Eat

A healthy diet that allows you to lose weight does not have to be boring in any sense. Try mixing ingredients, experiment with herbs and spices in the kitchen, create and taste. You will surprise yourself!

CHAPTER FIFTEEN

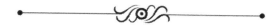

A 7 Day Kickstart Intermittent Fasting Weight Loss Plan for Women over 40

Every Doctor has their own opinions and solutions specifically suited to Women over 40, to help them to get the best out of their body during this period of great change within their body and especially in the run up towards Menopause.

Some of the methods that are recommended during this time of change to initiate weight loss are as follows:

Weightlifting

The body is starting to produce less estrogen; hence it is more difficult. Therefore, you must be able to lift weights to increase the level of metabolism and enhance your chances of losing weight.

Eat More Protein and Fiber:

Proteins help build muscle, reduce the feeling of hunger in the process. Protein does not store as much fat in the body; therefore, it helps build the body you desire even in your 40s.

Monitor Your Calories:

It works well if you are able to slowly monitor the intake of your calories and take the right steps to cut it back when needed. It is helpful to know when to cut back and decide exactly how much to reduce your intake with the help of your doctor.

Training Intervals

Doctors still agree that the best form of exercise are still cardiovascular exercises. High intense exercise could be carried out for 30 minutes five times a week to get started but check with your own healthcare provider to be sure if that is right for you.

Drink A Lot of Water

Often, it can be pretty difficult to remember that you have not taken in enough water, especially with the changes going on in your body. Therefore, you must be very deliberate about your water intake and take it at specific time intervals to stay hydrated. (I particularly like those water bottles with the markings on the side, so you can see exactly how much you have had)

Always remember that Losing weight and enjoying your best life is solely your responsibility and no one else's.

Everything you will ever need to live your life to the fullest is within your reach. Go for it!

The 7 Day Kickstart Intermittent Fasting Weight Loss Plan for Women over 40

The Following recipes are easily able to be scaled up or down as required, depending on the number of people, be it 2 ,4 or 1. Some people make a larger portion and will use the rest for a later meal.

With the Dinners these recipes are generally for 4 people, in an attempt to make it easier for families, for those not on the weight loss plan rice, noodles or potatoes can be added and those on the plan can have their meal with a simple green salad

These recipes can be easily mixed and matched and you can swop, one breakfast for another, one lunch for another or one Dinner for another, but do not swop mealtime options for each other- e.g., do not swop a Breakfast for a dinner, as the content of these recipes have been designed to give you the nutrients you need at various stages of the day and the best chance of weight loss success via Intermittent Fasting.

Day One

Breakfast: Spinach Parmesan Baked Eggs (Serves 2)

Ingredients

- Two teaspoons of olive oil

- Two cloves of garlic, chopped

- 4 cups of baby spinach

- 1/2 cup fat-free grated parmesan cheese

- Four eggs

- One small tomato, diced finely

Instructions

- Preheat the Oven to 350 degrees. Spray nonstick spray on an 8 inch by 8-inch casserole dish.

- Heat the olive oil in a large skillet over medium heat. Once hot, add the garlic and spinach. Sauté until the spinach is wilted. Remove any excess liquid from the heat and drain away. In the casserole dish, pour in the parmesan cheese and spoon the mixture into one even plate.

- For the eggs, make four tiny divots in the spinach. Crack each egg into a divot. Bake for 15 to 20 minutes, or until the majority of the egg whites are set. Remove from the oven and let the tomato cool for about 5 minutes, then sprinkle and Serve.

Lunch: Oven-Crisp Fish Tacos (Serves 2)

Ingredients

- 4 fish fillets cut into 2-inch strips (3 or 4 strips per fillet)

- ¼ cup of white, whole meal flour

- ¼ cup of corn flour

- ¼ cup of whole grain breadcrumbs

- Two tablespoons of freshly squeezed lime juice (1 medium-sized lime)

- Two tablespoons of taco seasoning,

- 4 (6 inches) corn tortillas or 4 (6 inches) whole wheat flour tortillas

- 1 cup of grated lettuce or cabbage

- 2 egg whites – lightly whisked

- 1 cup of salsa (without added sugar) or one medium-sized tomato, diced

- 1 cup of Greek-style fat-free yogurt, optionally fat-free sour cream

Instructions

- Oven preheated to 400 degrees F.

- Attach foil to a baking sheet. Place a cooling rack on top of the baking sheet and sprinkle with a spray of olive oil or canola oil.

- In a shallow bowl, mix the breadcrumbs, cornmeal, and taco seasoning.

- Whisk the egg whites and lime juice into a separate, shallow bowl until frothy.

- Place the flour into a shallow bowl.

- Gently dip the fish strips into the flour to coat lightly on both sides. dip in the whites of the eggs and allow excess to drip off, then push the fish pieces on both sides into the seasoned cornmeal and breadcrumbs.

- Place the breaded fish strips on the prepared rack and cook for 10 to 12 minutes until the golden crisp is on the outside and the fish is opaque and easily flakes with a fork.

- Coat with a cooking spray, a sauté pan, or skillet. Heat the tortillas over medium heat, for 30 seconds to 1 minute per side, until they cook. Hold the tortillas warm until ready to serve in a clean kitchen towel.

- Layer in each tortilla, top with shredded romaine, salsa or tomato, and yogurt.

Dinner: Easy Turkey Burrito Skillet (Serves 2)

Ingredients

- One tablespoon of chili powder

- 1/2 pound of ground turkey

- One teaspoon of ground cumin

- One tablespoon of lime juice

- 1/2 teaspoon of kosher salt

- 1/4 teaspoon of ground black pepper (or crushed Chili pepper if you like it spicy!)

- 1/4 cup of water

- 1 cup chunky salsa without sugar,

- One can of black beans, rinsed and drained

- 1 cup of low-fat cheddar cheese

- 1/2 cup of Greek yogurt

- 1/4 cup fresh coriander, chopped

Instructions

- Cook the ground turkey in a large skillet until it is cooked through, breaking the turkey into small pieces as it cooks. Stir in the powdered chili, cumin, lime juice, salt, pepper, water, salsa, and beans. Bring to a boil, and lower to a simmer. Simmer for three to five minutes, or until the sauce thickens.

- Remove from heat then cover with shredded cheese. Cover to melt the cheese. Top each serving with fresh cilantro and Greek yogurt. Serve with a green salad.

Day Two

Breakfast:

Hummus Breakfast Bowl (Serves 1- double quantity for 2 servings)

Ingredients

- 1 cup of cooked rice
- 4-5 frozen broccoli florets
- One large egg, soft-boiled or fried
- 2 tbsp hummus
- Pinch salt and pepper
- A pinch of sesame
- Sriracha to taste

Instructions

- Soft boil or fry one egg, making the yolk runny to provide the bowl with extra "sauce."
- While the egg is cooking, put the precooked rice and broccoli florets into a bowl with the and microwave for one minute on high, or until the rice is hot and the florets warm up.
- Add the hummus, fried egg, and a pinch of salt and pepper, add the rice and broccoli to the dish. Drizzle with sriracha and sprinkle on top with the sesame seeds.

Lunch:

Baked lemon salmon and asparagus foil packs (Serves 4)

Ingredients

- Four salmon fillets

- One lemon sliced

- One teaspoon of paprika

- One teaspoon of garlic powder

- One teaspoon of salt

- 1 tsp black pepper

- 1 pound of asparagus spears ends trimmed

- 1/2 cup of butter melted

- One lemon juiced

- One tablespoon of chopped garlic

- Two teaspoons of fresh basil

Garnish

- Fresh basil

- lemon slices

Instructions

1. Oven is preheated to 400 degrees.
2. Cut four strips of foil. 12x 18 centimeters, heavy foil.

3. Place two slices of lemon onto each foil pan.
4. Blend the paprika, garlic powder, salt, and pepper, and brush over the salmon.
5. Place each salmon filet in the lemon slices center.
6. Divide the asparagus into four equal portions and place on each piece of foil next to the salmon.
7. Blend the melted butter, lemon juice, garlic, and basil in a small bowl.
8. Garnish the butter mixture over each piece of salmon and asparagus.
9. Wrap the salmon and asparagus in foil, secure the edges to create a packet, and seal them.
10. Bake open foil packets in a preheated oven for 15-20 minutes and enjoy, or broil for 1-2 minutes to crisp, garnish with extra lemon juice and fresh basil and serve with a green salad.

Dinner: Chicken and Broccoli Stir Fry (Serves 4)

Ingredients

- 1 1/2 tablespoons peanut oil or coconut oil with a light taste,

- One medium-sized onion, cut into thin strips, approx. 1 1/2 cups

- Four cloves of garlic, chopped

- 1 pound of boneless skinless chicken cut into 2-inch pieces

- 1/2 teaspoon of cornstarch

- 1/3 cup low sodium soy sauce

- Two tablespoons of honey

- One tablespoon of chili paste

- 4 cups of broccoli florets

- boiled rice for serving, optional

Instructions

- Heat a large skillet over medium to high heat. Add a 1/2 tablespoon of oil and allow it to warm for a couple of seconds. Add the of the onion and allow to cook for 2 minutes. Add in the garlic and mix. Remove the garlic and onion from pan.

- Pour the remaining oil into the skillet center. Stir in the chicken. Allow the meat to begin to cook and sprinkle with cornstarch. Cook for 2 minutes without stirring until browned, then flip every piece of chicken. Cook for a further 1 minute, before beginning to add the other ingredients.

- While the chicken is cooking, mix the soy sauce, honey, and chili paste together. Apply the sauce to the pan and stir.

- In addition to the other ingredients, add the broccoli and cover the pan. Cook for another 2 minutes. The broccoli should be shiny green and barely soft. Remove the lid and stir, removing any bits of meat or sauce from the skillet's rim. Simmer for 1 more minute, frequently stirring to thicken the sauce. Serve over rice or alone, if desired.

Day Three

Breakfast: 4-Ingredient Protein Pancakes (Serves 1)

Ingredients

- 1 cup of oats

- One banana

- Two eggs

- Four teaspoons of baking powder

- a pinch of salt

- a pinch of cinnamon

- 1–2 scoops of protein powder

- Two tablespoons of flax flour

Instructions

- Run everything on medium-low speed through the blender until very well blended

- Heat a grid with a nonstick to medium-high heat. In small circles, add batter-about 1/4 cup per pancake. Sprinkle with raspberries or blueberries if you wish. When the edges start to look dry (2-3 minutes), flip on the other side and cook for another minute or two.

- Top with whatever you like! (I personally love mixed berries and flaked almonds with these)

-

Lunch: wild cod with Moroccan couscous (Serves 4)

Ingredients

- 1/2 cup chicken broth, fat-free, low in sodium

- One can of tomato cubes with green chili peppers

- One tablespoon and two teaspoons of extra virgin olive oil

- 1-1 1/2 cup Moroccan couscous (wholegrain couscous optional)

- Kosher or sea salt to taste

- Black pepper to taste

- 4 (4 ounces) wild-caught cod fillets,

- One tablespoon of freshly squeezed lemon juice

Instructions

- Add the couscous, chicken broth, two teaspoons of extra virgin olive oil, and diced tomatoes with juice in a medium saucepan. Switch to medium-high heat and bring couscous to a boil; add salt and pepper. Remove from heat, stir, then cover the saucepan, and leave the couscous to stand while cod is being prepared.

- Spice the cod with black pepper and sea salt. Add a tablespoon of oil to a large non-stick skillet, turn to a medium heat, and cook until the fish fillets on each side, for around 2-3 minutes, until they flake with a fork. Remove from the heat and serve with the couscous, Drizzle the juice of the lemon over the fillets just before serving.

Dinner: Honey & Garlic-Shrimp Stir Fry (Serves 4)

Ingredients

- Two tablespoons of rapeseed oil

- 1 pound of shrimp peeled & deveined

- Three cloves of chopped garlic

- 1 cup Snow Peas

- 2 cups of Bok Choy

- 1/4 cup honey

- Two tablespoons of lite soy sauce

- Sesame seeds optional

- Optional parsley

Instructions

1. In a non-stick skillet or wok add the oil on medium-high heat.
2. Add the shrimp and fry on each side for 1-2 minutes.
3. Remove the shrimp, add the garlic, and cook for 30 seconds.
4. Add the soy sauce and honey and whisk together.
5. Add the Snow peas & Bok Choy
6. Cook until reduced for 1 minute, then add the shrimp back to coat before serving, over rice or vegetables
7. Garnish and serve with parsley and sesame seeds.

Day Four

Breakfast:

Ham and Egg Breakfast skillet (Serves 2)

Ingredients

- 4 eggs

- 1/3 cup heavy whipped cream

- Cut 2/3 cup of ham into cubes

- 1/2 green onion, chopped

- Splash of salt

- Pinch of pepper

- Four teaspoons of butter

- 4 ounces of cream cheese, diced

Instructions

1. Whisk the eggs and the cream in a large bowl; stir in ham, onion, salt, and pepper, and heat butter over medium heat in a large skillet. Add the egg mixture   stir and cook until almost set. Add cream cheese, stir and Cook until set before serving.

Lunch:

Sweet Potato and Turkey Skillet (Serves 2)

Ingredients

- One tablespoon of extra virgin olive oil

- One medium onion, chopped

- One teaspoon of cumin

- 1/2-pound lean ground turkey

- Two medium-sized sweet potatoes, cut into small cubes

- Two fresh sage leaves, roughly chopped

- 1/2 teaspoon of kosher or sea salt

- 1/4 teaspoon of pepper

- 1/2 cup partially skimmed mozzarella, grated

Directions

- Over a medium-low heat, sauté the onion in a large pan with extra virgin olive oil until tender, about 4 minutes. Add the turkey, mix cook it is not pink anymore. Drain away ant excess fat. Stir in the sweet potatoes, cumin, garlic, salt, pepper. Stir and cook for about 5-10 minutes until the sweet potatoes are tender but do not fall apart.

- Sprinkle the mozzarella over when the sweet potatoes are tender, cover, then turn off the heat.

- Wait until the cheese melts before serving.

Dinner: Savory Lemon White Fish Fillets

Ingredients

- 4 (4 to 6 ounces) white fish fillets

- Three tablespoons of olive oil, divided

- 1/4 teaspoon of kosher or sea salt

- 1/4 tsp freshly ground black pepper

- Two lemons, one halved, one cut into wedges

Instructions

- Allow the fish to sit for 10-15 minutes in a bowl at room temperature.

- Apply a spoonful of olive oil and sprinkle salt and pepper on either side of each fillet. Place a skillet or pan over medium heat and add two spoonful's of olive oil. Add the fish after about one minute, when the oil is hot and shimmering but not smoking. Cook on each side for two to three minutes so that the fish is browned on each side and cooked through.

- Squeeze both halves of lemon over the fish and remove them from heat. If any lemon juice is left in the pan, pour it over the fish before serving. Serve with wedges of Lemon and a green salad.

Day Five

Breakfast:

Sweet Potato Breakfast Hash (Serves 2)

Ingredients

- One teaspoon of avocado oil or coconut oil,

- One large onion, chopped

- One sweet bell pepper, diced

- 2 large tomatoes diced

- Two large, sweet potatoes, peeled and cut into ¾ inch cubes

- ½ cup of chicken or vegetable broth

- One teaspoon of coarse kosher salt

- ½ teaspoon of smoked paprika

- ½ teaspoon of Italian spice

- ¼ teaspoon of garlic powder

- ¼ teaspoon of ground pepper or to taste

Instructions

- Heat 1 tablespoon oil over medium-high heat in a large, non-stick skillet. Add the onion, tomatoes and pepper and cook for about 4 to 5 minutes, frequently stirring until the onion just starts to brown. Add sweet potatoes and cook for further 6 minutes, frequently stirring, until the sweet potatoes brown in a few places.

148

- Add the broth and cover, then bring to a simmer. Reduce heat to medium-low and keep simmering until the sweet potatoes begin to soften, around 12 minutes, removing the lid to stir.

- Add the remaining one teaspoon of oil to coat and stir. Stir frequently and add paprika, Italian seasoning, garlic powder, and ground pepper. Let the hash cook, stir until crispy and brown in spots and the sweet potatoes are soft enough to break down in half easily when tested with a spatula, after about 6 minutes.

- Serve hot or cool, and keep for up to 5 days in a resealable container, alternatively you can upgrade this recipe to lunch by adding chicken breast

Lunch:

Chicken Breast, Zucchini and Snow Pea stir fry (Serves 2)

Ingredients

- One tablespoon of peanut oil

- One teaspoon of sesame oil

- One medium onion, chopped

- One 1/2 to one teaspoon of chili flakes

- 1 clove of garlic

- 1/2-pound Chicken Breast strips

- 1 medium zucchini, cut into small cubes

- 2 cups of snow peas

149

- Two fresh sage leaves, roughly chopped

- 1/2 teaspoon of kosher or sea salt

- 1/4 teaspoon of pepper

- Sesame seeds to garnish

Directions

1. Over medium-low heat, sauté the onion in a large saucepan with the oil until tender, about 2-3 minutes. Add the chicken strips, stir until cooked. Drain away any excess fat. Stir in the zucchini, garlic, and the dry ingredients continue to cook for a further 2 mins before adding in the snow peas and the sesame oil and continue to Stir and cook for a further 2-3 mins.

2. Add the chicken back in stir and incorporate all the ingredients and turn off the heat.

3. Serve with a garnish of Sesame Seeds

Dinner:

Salmon Parcels (Serves 4)

Ingredients

- Pre heat the Oven to 400 degrees

- Grease proof oven paper or foil for the parcels, cut into strips big enough, to accommodate the fillets

- 4 (4 to 6 ounces) Salmon Fillets

- Three tablespoons of olive oil, divided

- 1/4 teaspoon of kosher or sea salt

- 1 tablespoon of Melted Butter

- 1/4 tsp freshly ground black pepper

- 1 teaspoon dill plus some for garnish

- Two lemons, one halved, one cut into wedges

Instructions

- Mix the dill with a tablespoonful of melted butter and add salt and pepper to this before brushing each Salmon Fillet with the mixture. Place each Salmon Fillet onto lemon slices on the oven the paper before sealing the parcels for the oven.

- Bake for parcels in a preheated oven for 15 mins garnish with extra lemon juice and Dill before serving with a green salad and with wedges of Lemon.

Day Six

Breakfast:

Scrambled eggs with lox (Serves 2)

Ingredients

- Six eggs
- Butter
- ½ tablespoon Lite Olive Oil
- 1 Tablespoon of Heavy Cream
- Strips of lox
- 1 teaspoon of Dill
- 1 teaspoon of fresh Parsley
- Salt & Pepper to taste
- Wedges of Lemon

Instructions

1. Whisk the eggs softly with a fork
2. Heat a nonstick pan on a low heat.
3. Add the Butter to melt and the pan and the lite olive oil to the pan to prevent the Butter from burning one the Butter has melted add the eggs to the pan followed by the Dill and fold in as the eggs begin to cook add in the cream.
4. Add the lox and continue to stir gently
5. Add Salt and pepper to taste and as the eggs look as though they are about to set remove from the heat and serve garnished with Fresh Parsley and a wedge of Lemon.

Lunch:

Pesto Chicken wraps (Serves 2)

Ingredients

- 2 Chicken Breasts

- ½ Cup Pesto

- 2 large Tortilla Wraps

- 1 Sweet pepper – cut into thin strips

- Shredded lettuce

- 2 Tablespoons of low-fat flavored Mayo of your choice

Instructions

- Preheat the Oven to 350 degrees

- Brush both sides of the Chicken with the Pesto and place in a baking dish and cook in the Oven for 12-15 mins.

- Remove the chicken from the Oven when cooked and allow to cool before cutting into strips.

- Spread the Tortillas with the Mayo, layer with the lettuce and sweet peppers and chicken and wrap to serve, if you want to enjoy these without the wrap just serve in a bowl.

Dinner:

Sweet Chili Shrimp Stir Fry (Serves 4)

Ingredients

- Two tablespoons of rapeseed oil
- 1 pound of shrimp peeled & deveined
- 2 cloves of garlic chopped
- 4 cups of Bok Choy
- 2 cups of Baby corn
- 1/4 cup honey
- 1 tablespoon sweet chilis
- 1 sweet pepper
- Two tablespoons of lite soy sauce
- Sesame seeds optional
- Optional parsley

Instructions

- In a non-stick skillet or wok, add the oil on medium-high heat.
- Add the shrimp and cook gently on each side for 1-2 minutes.
- Remove the shrimp, add the garlic, and cook for 30 seconds.
- Add the Baby Corn, pepper, the sweet chilies and allow to cook for a further 2 mins before adding the Bok Choy.

- Mix the soy sauce and honey before adding to the pan.

- Cook until reduced for 1 minute, and then add the shrimp back to coat before serving

- Garnish, with parsley and sesame seeds and serve as desired.

Day Seven

Breakfast

Breakfast: Spanish Baked Eggs (Serves 2)

Ingredients

- Two teaspoons of olive oil

- Two cloves of garlic, chopped

- 4 cups of fresh tomatoes (put some aside for garnish)

- 1 can of tinned tomatoes

- 1/2 cup fat-free grated parmesan cheese

- Four eggs

- Salt & Pepper to taste

- 1/2 Cup Fresh Parsley

Instructions

- Oven pre-heated to 350 degrees. Spray nonstick spray on an 8 inch by 8-inch casserole dish.

- Heat the olive oil in a large skillet over medium heat. Once hot, add the garlic and tomatoes (tinned and fresh). Sauté until the tomatoes are beginning to soften and add Salt and Pepper to taste

- Add the mixture to the casserole dish and make 4 little divots, crack the eggs into the divots and sprinkle parmesan cheese over the top.

- Cook in the Oven for 12-15 mins, until the whites of the eggs are set,

- Remove from the Oven and allow to Cool for 5 mins

- Sprinkle with Parsley and Serve.

Lunch:

Chicken Tacos (Serves 2)

Ingredients

1. 2 Chicken Breast Fillets,
2. Two tablespoons of freshly squeezed lime or Lemon juice (1 medium-sized lime or Lemon)
3. Two tablespoons of taco seasoning, the recipe for homemade taco seasoning
4. 4(6 inches) corn tortillas or 4 (6 inches) whole wheat flour tortillas
5. 1 cup of grated lettuce or cabbage
6. 1 cup of salsa (without added sugar) or one medium-sized tomato, diced
7. 1 cup of Greek-style fat-free yogurt, optionally fat-free sour cream

Instructions

- Oven preheats to 450 degrees F.

- Attach foil to a baking sheet. Place a cooling rack on top of the baking sheet and sprinkle with a spray of olive oil or canola oil.

- On a shallow plate, massage the taco seasoning into the chicken breasts.

157

- Coat a baking tray with a cooking spray

- Place the Chicken breasts on the baking tray and bake in the oven for about 12-15 mins until cooked,

- Remove from the oven and allow to cool

- Shred the chicken breasts using the 2-fork method.

- Layer each tortilla with the chicken and top with shredded lettuce/cabbage salsa or tomato, and yogurt.

Dinner:

Easy Steak and Vegetable Bowl (Serves 4)

Ingredients

- 1 pound Steak (cut into thin Strips)

- 2 cups of sweet peppers

- One cup Onions

- One cup Spinach

- One Cup of Broccoli

- Two cups' Mushrooms

- One tablespoon of Mixed Herbs

- One tablespoon of chili powder

- 1/2 Cup of Fresh Parsley

- One tablespoon of lime juice

- 1/2 teaspoon of kosher salt

- 1/4 teaspoon of ground black pepper (or crushed red pepper if you like it spicy!)

- 1/4 cup of water

Instructions

- Brown the Steak strips in a large non skillet until they begin to cook,

- Remove the steak from the pan and add the onions to the pan to soften

- Add in the Broccoli Cook for one min before adding the water and the other vegetables, apart from the mushrooms

- Add all the dry ingredients in and mix well, so that everything is coated.

- Add the steak back in together with the mushrooms making sure that everything is well coated and cook for a further 2 mins.

- Serve with a Garnish of Fresh Parsley and a squeeze of lime, over Rice or as it is in a Bowl.

CONCLUSION

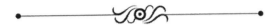

For women over 40, who are interested in weight loss, This Book will have clearly shown that Intermittent Fasting appears to be a really good option and will provide substantial other health benefits as well.

This Book has covered a lot of ground both from a general information perspective around Intermittent Fasting as well as a huge amount of Specific Information relevant to Women over 40, (towards who this book was aimed) and more specifically how Intermittent Fasting relates to them and the changes going on in the female body around this age, as the female body begins its transition to prepare for the changes leading to menopause. We have looked at a variety of types of Intermittent Fasting methods and what might suit you best. We have also looked at how best to implement it to accelerate weight loss and in addition we have looked at Superfoods and powerful anti-ageing foods as well as the best exercises to do for Women Over 40.

In addition, there is also a 7 Day Kickstart Intermittent Fasting Weight Loss Plan for Women over 40.

However, most people still want to know whether it is beneficial to them.

Is intermittent fasting beneficial to females?

Clearly it is incredibly beneficial for many, but there are also some women for whom it is unsuitable and some of those instances have been mentioned in this book already.

However, it needs to be stressed that your Medical Practitioner should always be consulted before embarking on any program of this kind to clearly establish if it is a viable option for you as an individual.

A number of primary studies on intermittent fasting have been published, and they can help shed some light on this fascinating and increasingly popular new dietary trend, (although it must be noted that Intermittent fasting is not a New trend and that it has been around for thousands of years).

There are several variations on this diet, Intermittent fasting is also known as alternate-day fasting. Research published in the American Journal of Clinical Nutrition recently enrolled a number of obese men and women in a 10-week program. On fasting days, participants ate up to 25% of their estimated energy requirements. They were given dietary advice for the remainder of the period but no clear guidelines to follow.

The participants did lose weight as planned as a result of the study, but the researchers were even more interested in some particular improvements. After just ten weeks, the participants were all still obese, but their cholesterol, LDL-cholesterol, triglycerides, and systolic blood pressure had all markedly improved. As further studies continued, the fact that many participants still even had more weight to lose than the original study participants before getting the same results made this an even more fascinating discovery. It was this remarkable discovery that has inspired many people to begin to pursue fasting.

Intermittent fasting undoubtedly has some benefits for women. The fact that women have a much higher fat proportion in their bodies makes it particularly relevant for women who are trying to lose weight. When attempting to lose weight, the body burns carbohydrate reserves for the first 6 hours before transitioning to fat burning. Fasting is a viable option for women who are still dealing with stubborn fat despite maintaining a balanced diet and a healthy exercise schedule.

Obviously, there is a general correlation between our emotional development and our physical changes as our bodies begin to transition towards and go through menopause. One of the most important changes that women over 40 will undergo is that their metabolism slows down, which leads to the accumulation of body fat around the center of their figure. Whilst restricting calorie intake can help with fat loss, this pattern of intermittent fasting has been shown to help control hunger and result in better diet adherence in the long term. If you are a woman over 40, you should try intermittently fasting to keep from eating more than your body needs on a regular basis and help it acclimate to a slowing metabolism.

Cholesterol and high blood pressure are also applied to the list of chronic disorders that are present in many adults. While intermittent fasting has been shown to decrease both total cholesterol and blood pressure, it has been noticeable in a variety of studies that not all that much weight loss is required to achieve good results. Researchers are still exploring to find out whether there are other benefits of intermittent fasting without so much weight loss. If you've managed to stop the increase in your weight at the doctor's office, you might be able to help your other adverse physiological numbers through losing a little weight or by medical measures.

It is clear, that while Intermittent Fasting has undoubted benefits, to improve health and accelerate weight loss especially in women over 40 years of age, Intermittent fasting is not appropriate for every woman and your Medical professional should be consulted as a matter of course before embarking on any kind of regime for weight loss. especially if you have any underlying Health concerns, to ensure that it is an appropriate option for you.